Teaching and Learning Oncology Communication

Jack Pun
Editor

Teaching and Learning Oncology Communication

A Cross-Disciplinary Perspectives in Chinese Context

Springer

Editor
Jack Pun
Department of English
The Chinese University of Hong Kong
Hong Kong SAR, China

ISBN 978-981-96-9473-0 ISBN 978-981-96-9474-7 (eBook)
https://doi.org/10.1007/978-981-96-9474-7

This Springer imprint is published by the registered company Springer Nature Singapore Pte Ltd.
The registered company address is: 152 Beach Road, #21-01/04 Gateway East, Singapore 189721, Singapore

For patients and their families, and the frontline healthcare professionals who strive every day to navigate the complexities of communication with empathy, clarity, and cultural sensitivity, fostering understanding and trust during some of life's most challenging conversations.

Acknowledgements

This book would not have been possible without the collective efforts and unwavering support of numerous individuals and institutions who have contributed to its development. First, I would like to express my deepest gratitude to the healthcare professionals, educators, and researchers whose insights and expertise have enriched this volume. Your dedication to advancing oncology communication within the Chinese context has been a profound source of inspiration. I extend my heartfelt thanks to the patients and families who shared their stories, experiences, and challenges. Your voices remind me of the importance of compassionate and effective communication in healthcare.

Special recognition goes to the interdisciplinary team of contributors who brought their diverse perspectives to this book. I am grateful to the many thoughtful and constructive suggestions we received from our colleagues and collaborators, which have had a significant impact on the content of the included chapters. Your commitment to bridging the fields of oncology, linguistics, medical education, and cross-cultural studies has made this endeavour truly unique. Special thanks to Ms. Kexin Tan (Casey) for her support in preparing this book as well as the conclusion chapter. I would like to thank all the reviewers, whose comments and useful suggestions greatly enhanced the quality of this edited volume. Also, I would like to express sincere gratitude to the staff at Springer, especially for Mr. Rajasekar Ganesan and Ms. Melody Zhang, for guiding me through and assisting with the editing process from start to finish.

To my readers—healthcare practitioners, educators, policymakers, and students—this book is dedicated to you. It is my hope that these pages serve as a valuable resource in improving communication practices and fostering greater understanding and collaboration in oncology care. Thank you all for being part of this collaborative effort to enhance the teaching and learning of oncology communication in the Chinese context.

Contents

Editor and Contributors

About the Editor

Jack Pun is Associate Professor in the Department of English at the Chinese University of Hong Kong, Hong Kong SAR, China. He completed his Ph.D. at the University of Oxford. As a bilingual speaker of Chinese and English, he is motivated to investigate the effectiveness and patient satisfaction of health communication from a cross-cultural and cross-disciplinary perspective. He explores the role of communication in shaping decision making processes at consultations, and how communication affects the quality of care patients received from the health providers in different clinical settings (emergency department, intensive care unit, nursing handovers, traditional Chinese medicine, veterinary medicine) and how effective communication enhances our understanding of the challenges and expectations in healthcare in worldwide hospital setting. *He is a founding member of the Institute for Communication in Healthcare (ICH) at the Australian National University, ANU, Canberra, Australia.* He is associate editor of *Journal of Research in Science & Technological Education*, and published a recent monograph, *the Role of Language in Eastern and Western Health communication by Routledge.*

Contributors

Tsz Yeung Kam Hong Kong, China

Sunny Kong Department of Medicine, Hong Kong Buddhist Hospital, Hong Kong, China

Weiwei Lu Department of Social and Behavioural Sciences, City University of Hong Kong, Hong Kong, China

Jack Pun Department of English, The Chinese University of Hong Kong, Hong Kong SAR, China

Kexin Tan Department of English and Communication, The Hong Kong Polytechnic University, Hong Kong SAR, China

Qianwen Joyce Yu School of Foreign Languages, Soochow University, Suzhou, China

Chapter 1
Introduction

Jack Pun

Introduction

Healthcare in Hong Kong Special Administrative Region (SAR), China, is characterised by a unique mixture of Western and Chinese values, offering a distinctive basis for evaluating cross-cultural expectations, practices, and experiences in clinical communication. Over the past decade, there has been a growing interest in examining the role of clinical communication, particularly in the context of oncology, within the Chinese setting (Pun et al., 2020). This book aims to address the gap in understanding how oncology communication functions in this specific Chinese context and to develop culturally appropriate models that improve the clinician-patient relationship (Pun & Wong, 2022).

In China, significant differences in beliefs and practices arise during clinical encounters compared to the West. Many clinicians trained in Hong Kong are familiar with English-speaking, Western-based communication frameworks but often face challenges when interacting with patients and caregivers in their mother tongue, Cantonese (Pun, 2021a, 2022, 2023). Traditional Chinese philosophies, which regard death as a taboo subject, further complicate these interactions, making clinicians hesitant to discuss crucial topics such as prognosis, Advanced Care Planning (ACP), or organ donation (Pun, 2021b). These cultural influences have led to a persistent gap in recognizing the importance of effective communication in the face of serious terminal illnesses (Pun et al., 2021; Pun et al., 2023).

Western models of healthcare communication, while widely adopted, do not seamlessly translate to the Chinese context (Zhou & Nunes, 2016). There is an urgent need to develop communication strategies that are culturally sensitive and adapted to local values and practices (Pun et al., 2018). This book, therefore, proposes the development of a Chinese-specific oncology communication model, which could bridge this

J. Pun (✉)
Department of English, The Chinese University of Hong Kong, Hong Kong SAR, China
e-mail: jackpun@cuhk.edu.hk

J. Pun (ed.), *Teaching and Learning Oncology Communication*,
https://doi.org/10.1007/978-981-96-9474-7_1

gap and foster better communication between clinicians and cancer patients. This volume brings together diverse perspectives from the sharing of key stakeholders in oncology care, including oncologists, palliative care specialists, nurses, counsellors, cancer patients, and health communication experts. By drawing on insights from multiple disciplines, the book seeks to offer a comprehensive view of oncology communication in the Chinese context and provide guidance for teaching and practising effective communication in this field (Pun & Chor, 2020; Pun et al., 2015, 2016).

The Role of Oncology Communication in the Chinese Context

Healthcare in Hong Kong and Mainland China presents a unique fusion of Western medical practices and deeply ingrained Chinese cultural values. This blend creates a distinctive environment for oncology communication, where cross-cultural expectations and practices influence clinical interactions. This book, *Teaching and LearningOncology Communication—A Cross-disciplinary Perspective in theChinese Context*, seeks to explore the complexities of oncology communication in this setting, highlighting the need for culturally appropriate strategies that better serve both clinicians and patients.

In the Chinese cultural context, communication around cancer care is shaped by traditional philosophies and family-centric decision-making processes, which often complicate clinician-patient interactions (Pun et al., 2021). In Hong Kong, many clinicians are trained using Western-based communication frameworks, typically emphasizing patient autonomy and open disclosure. However, these practices do not always translate effectively in the Chinese context, where families often prefer to shield the patient from distressing news, especially regarding terminal illness or end-of-life care (Pun et al., 2023). This cultural clash presents a significant challenge in oncology communication, particularly in dealing with topics like advanced care planning (ACP), organ donation, and discussing prognosis (Pun, 2021b). This introduction chapter will outline the overarching themes of the book, present the key challenges in oncology communication in Chinese settings, and preview the structure and focus of the subsequent chapters.

Oncology Communication in Chinese Healthcare

Oncology communication is a critical aspect of cancer care that encompasses the delivery of diagnoses, treatment plans, prognoses, and end-of-life care discussions (Back et al., 2008). In Western contexts, open and honest communication is regarded as essential to patient-centered care. However, in Chinese culture, where death is often considered a taboo subject, conversations about terminal illness are frequently avoided (Cheng et al., 2019; Xu, 2007). This reluctance stems from the deeply embedded Chinese cultural values of maintaining hope and emotional stability within the family unit, as well as the desire to protect patients from emotional harm.

As review in the chapter 2, Chinese philosophies on life and death, the concept of a "good death," and the critical role of family in decision-making are central to how patients and their caregivers perceive medical information. In many cases, families take on a protective role, making decisions on behalf of the patient, particularly in end-of-life situations. This contrasts sharply with Western notions of individual autonomy, creating an ethical tension for clinicians who must balance the family's wishes with the patient's right to know about their health status.

The need for culturally adapted communication strategies becomes especially apparent when dealing with sensitive issues such as delivering bad news, as discussed in Chapter 4, the use of direct language in Western medical communication often needs to be softened or replaced with more nuanced approaches in Chinese settings to align with cultural expectations of tact and indirectness. The chapter also discusses how healthcare professionals can navigate these challenges by adapting the SPIKES protocol—a structured approach to breaking bad news—to the Chinese cultural context.

Cultural Influences on Oncology Communication

Chinese culture places a strong emphasis on family roles and the concept of relational autonomy, where the family often serves as the primary decision-maker for the patient. As detailed in Chapter 7, Confucian values continue to shape medical decision-making, especially in palliative and end-of-life care. The deference to family members can lead to ethical dilemmas for clinicians who may be asked to withhold information from the patient at the family's request. While this is done out of a desire to protect the patient from distress, it raises important questions about patient autonomy and informed consent.

Furthermore, traditional Chinese beliefs surrounding death—such as the reluctance to discuss terminal illness—often delay crucial conversations about prognosis and end-of-life care. Chapter 6 examines how cultural norms influence the timing and content of prognostic discussions. Patients in Chinese settings may not always be informed of their terminal status, as families prefer to shield them from the emotional burden. This chapter highlights the importance of prognostication in palliative care and the challenges clinicians face in providing culturally sensitive yet transparent information to patients and their families.

The Role of Traditional Chinese Medicine (TCM)

Another layer of complexity in oncology communication arises from the integration of Traditional Chinese Medicine (TCM) into cancer care. TCM is deeply rooted in Chinese cultural beliefs and often viewed as a holistic complement to Western medical treatments. Patients may choose to combine or alternate between Western and TCM approaches, which can create challenges for clinicians in communicating treatment plans and managing patient expectations (Pun & Wong, 2022). Chapter 3 explores how oncologists navigate these dual medical paradigms. Clinicians must respect patients' cultural preferences for TCM while ensuring that treatments are evidence-based and effective.

The inclusion of TCM in cancer care adds another dimension to the communication process, as patients may prioritize TCM's focus on long-term well-being and harmony over immediate clinical outcomes. Oncologists, therefore, need to engage in sensitive conversations that respect these beliefs while guiding patients towards medically sound decisions. This challenge underscores the need for interdisciplinary collaboration between oncologists, TCM practitioners, and other healthcare professionals to provide integrated care that aligns with both cultural values and medical efficacy.

A Multidisciplinary Approach to Oncology Communication

This book takes a multidisciplinary approach to understanding oncology communication in the Chinese context. As highlighted in Chapter 2, this approach involves contributions from oncologists, palliative care specialists, nurses, counsellors, and TCM practitioners, all of whom play key roles in shaping patient care. By incorporating diverse perspectives, the book aims to provide a holistic understanding of the communication challenges at each stage of the cancer care journey.

From the initial diagnosis to palliative care and end-of-life discussions, oncology communication must be tailored to the unique needs of Chinese patients. The chapters that follow offer practical insights into how healthcare professionals can navigate the cultural and ethical complexities of oncology communication. For example, Chapter 3 examines how oncologists in Chinese hospitals construct their professional identities while managing the demands of cancer care, highlighting the importance of empathy, cultural sensitivity, and interdisciplinary collaboration.

The Aims of This Book

- **Objective 1: Understanding the Chinese Perspective in Oncology Communication** We delve into the cultural attitudes and beliefs that shape oncology communication in Chinese context. It examines how Chinese cultural values, such as the avoidance of death-related conversations and the importance of family involvement, influence patient interactions and decision-making.
- **Objective 2: Case Studies from the Chinese Clinical Context** We presents real-world case studies from Chinese oncology settings, illustrating the challenges and successes of communication in diverse clinical environments. These case studies offer valuable insights into how clinicians navigate cultural barriers and provide practical examples of culturally sensitive communication strategies.
- **Objective 3: Closing the Gap in Oncology Communication** We discuss strategies for improving oncology communication in Chinese context. It features contributions from practitioners who have developed innovative approaches to overcoming cultural obstacles and enhancing patient outcomes. This section emphasizes the need for ongoing education and training for healthcare professionals to develop the cultural competence necessary for effective communication in Chinese oncology care.

The Structure of This Book

This book provides comprehensive exploration of the cultural, linguistic, and professional dimensions of oncology communication within the Chinese cultural framework. This interdisciplinary volume draws on contributions from oncologists, palliative care specialists, health communication experts, and researchers to provide insights into the unique challenges and opportunities of clinical communication in Chinese oncology settings.

At its core, the book underscores the significance of culturally sensitive communication strategies in enhancing patient-centered care and fostering trust between healthcare providers, patients, and families. It addresses the complexities of integrating traditional Chinese values, such as family-centric decision-making and the reluctance to openly discuss terminal illnesses, with modern medical practices. Through in-depth analysis and case studies, the volume emphasizes the need for healthcare professionals to develop cultural competence and adapt Western communication models to align with local beliefs and practices.

Key themes include the role of family in oncology communication, the impact of cultural norms on prognostication and end-of-life care, and the ethical dilemmas that arise when balancing patient autonomy with family expectations. The book also highlights practical communication frameworks, such as adapting the SPIKES protocol, to navigate sensitive discussions about diagnosis, treatment, and advanced care planning in Chinese settings.

The volume is structured around pivotal topics:

- **Introduction**: Establishes the foundation by highlighting the unique cultural and linguistic aspects of oncology communication in Hong Kong and Mainland China, offering a contextual backdrop for the discussions to follow.
- **Cultural Contexts and Challenges**: Explores traditional Chinese philosophies on life, death, and family involvement in medical decision-making, examining the tensions between Eastern and Western approaches to healthcare.
- **Professional Identity and Communication**: Investigates how oncologists navigate their professional identities within the sociocultural expectations of their roles, emphasizing the impact of these dynamics on clinical interactions.
- **Breaking Bad News**: Analyzes the importance of culturally and linguistically sensitive strategies for delivering bad news, adapting established frameworks like the SPIKES protocol to resonate with Chinese cultural norms.
- **Prognostication in Palliative Care**: Discusses the intricate processes of estimating and communicating life expectancy, addressing ethical and cultural complexities that shape these interactions in the Chinese context.
- **End-of-Life Communication**: Focuses on the essential role of dignity and shared decision-making in facilitating a "good death," aligning with Chinese cultural values and familial priorities.
- **Family Dynamics in Oncology Communication**: Utilizes case studies to illustrate the significant influence of family members in treatment decisions, diagnosis disclosure, and end-of-life care, highlighting the importance of their role in Chinese settings.
- **Conclusion**: Reflects on the overarching lessons learned, advocating for greater interdisciplinary collaboration, culturally informed policy development, and community engagement to enhance oncology communication practices in Chinese healthcare systems.

Conclusion

As the cancer burden continues to rise globally, particularly in Hong Kong, there is an urgent need to develop communication models that respect cultural values while promoting effective patient care. This book aims to bridge the gap between Western-based communication frameworks and the unique cultural context of Chinese oncology patients. By offering both theoretical perspectives and practical case studies, the book provides a comprehensive guide to improving oncology communication in Chinese context. Healthcare professionals, educators, and researchers will find this volume an invaluable resource for understanding the cultural complexities of oncology communication in the Chinese context. Ultimately, this book serves as a call to action for the development of culturally informed communication strategies that enhance the clinician-patient relationship and improve patient outcomes in cancer care

Discussion Prompts

1 What are the main cultural challenges identified in the chapter regarding oncology communication in the Chinese context?
2 How do Chinese beliefs about death and family involvement contrast with Western principles of medical ethics and communication?
3 In what ways might Traditional Chinese Medicine (TCM) influence the communication between patients and healthcare professionals?
4 How do the communication models discussed in the chapter attempt to bridge the gap between Western frameworks and Chinese cultural values?
5 What role should interdisciplinary collaboration play in developing effective oncology communication in Hong Kong and Mainland China?

Reflection Questions

1 Which aspect of culturally sensitive communication in oncology did you find most relevant or surprising, and why?
2 Think about your own cultural background: How might it influence your expectations around healthcare communication, particularly in serious illness contexts?
3 How can healthcare professionals be trained to recognize and respect cultural differences while still ensuring ethical and patient-centered care?
4 What steps could be taken in policy or clinical practice to better integrate family roles without compromising patient autonomy?
5 How might this chapter inform your own approach to communication—whether as a researcher, educator, or practitioner—in a multicultural healthcare environment?

References

Back, A. L., Anderson, W. G., Bunch, L., Marr, L. A., Wallace, J. A., Yang, H. B., & Arnold, R. M. (2008). Communication about cancer near the end of life. *Cancer, 113*(S7), 1897–1910.
Cheng, H. W. B., Shek, P. S. K., Man, C. W., Chan, O. M., Chan, C. H., Lai, K. M., Cheng, S. C., Fung, K. S., Lui, W. K., Lam, C., Ng, Y. K., Wong, W. T., & Wong, C. (2019). Dealing with death taboo: Discussion of do-not-resuscitate directives with Chinese patients with noncancer life-limiting illnesses. *American Journal of Hospice and Palliative Medicine®, 36*(9), 760–766.
Pun, J. (2021a). Clinical handover in a bilingual setting: Interpretative phenomenological analysis to explore translanguaging practices for effective communication among hospital staff. *British Medical Journal Open, 11*(9), Article e046494. https://doi.org/10.1136/bmjopen-2020-046494
Pun, J. (2021b). Communication about advance directives and advance care planning in the East Asian context: A systematic review. *Oncology Nursing Forum, 49*(1), 58–70.
Pun, J. (2022). The priorities, challenges, and scope of clinical communication teaching perceived by clinicians from different disciplines: A Hong Kong case study. *BMC Primary Care, 22*(158), 1–16.
Pun, J. (2023). *The role of language in Eastern and Western health communication.* Routledge.

Pun, J., & Chor, W. (2020). Use of questioning between traditional Chinese medicine practitioners and patients to realize TCM philosophy: Holism, five elements and Yin-Yang in the context of Doctor–Patient communication. *Health Communication, 37*(2), 163–176.

Pun, J. C., Cheung, K. M. & Chow, C. H. J. (2021). A systematic review of teaching end of life communication: The priorities, the challenges and the scope. *BMJ Supportive & Palliative Care, 12*(4), 368–375.

Pun, J., Cheung, K. M., Chow, C. H. J., & Chan, W.L. (2020). Chinese perspective on end-of-life communication: A systematic review. *BMJ Supportive & Palliative Care, 14*(e1), e30-e37.

Pun, J., & Wong, W. (2022). Navigating communication between conventional medicine and traditional Chinese medicine: A case study of cancer patients in Hong Kong. *Supportive Care in Cancer, 30*(7), 5729–5735.

Pun, J., Chan, E. A., Wang, S., & Slade, D. (2018). Health professional-patient communication practices in East Asia: An integrative review of an emerging field of research and practice in Hong Kong, South Korea, Japan, Taiwan, and Mainland China. *Patient Education and Counseling., 101*(7), 1193–1206.

Pun, J., Chow, J. C. H., Fok, L., & Cheung, K. M. (2023). The role of patients' family members in end-of-life communication: An Integrative review. *BMJ Open, 13*(2).

Pun, J., Matthiessen, C. M. I. M., Slade, D., & Murray, K. (2015). Factors affecting communication in emergency departments: Doctors and nurses' perceptions of communication in a trilingual ED in Hong Kong. *International Journal of Emergency Medicine, 8*, 48.

Pun, K. H. J., Chan, E. A., Murray, K. A., Slade, D., & Matthiessen, C. M. I. M. (2016). Complexities of emergency communication: Clinicians' perceptions of communication challenges in a trilingual emergency department. *Journal of Clinical Nursing, 26*(21–22), 3396–3407. https://doi.org/10.1111/jocn.13699

Xu, Y. (2007). Death and dying in the Chinese culture: Implications for health care practice. *Home Health Care Management & Practice, 19*(5), 412–414.

Zhou, L., & Nunes, M. B. (2016). Barriers to knowledge sharing in Chinese healthcare referral services: An emergent theoretical model. *Global Health Action, 9*(1), 29964.

Chapter 2
Talking with Chinese Patients About Cancer—What Do We Know?

Jack Pun

Introduction

Effective clinical communication in oncology context is critical to delivering good patient-centred care, particularly in contexts where cultural values significantly influence how cancer is understood and discussed (Tay et al., 2017). In Hong Kong, where traditional values and philosophies continue to shape societal views on life, death, and illness, oncology communication presents unique communication challenges (Chan et al., 2018; Pun et al., 2018). Chinese cultural norms, especially regarding the role of the family in patient care, philosophies surrounding death, and the concept of a "good death," necessitate a distinct approach compared to the Western clinical models (Fu & Glasdam, 2022; Wang et al., 2020). This chapter seeks to review the current body of literature on oncology communication, particularly with Chinese patients in Chinese context, with a focus on understanding the cultural priorities that shape these interactions. By examining studies from various stages of clinical settings in oncology, we aim to highlight how Chinese philosophies on life and death, the importance of family involvement, and the cultural perception of terminal illness inform the communication between clinicians and patients (Dong et al., 2016).

This chapter begins with an exploration of key cultural elements such as the traditional reluctance to discuss death and the preference for family-centred decision-making in the Chinese context. From there, it evaluates the existing literature on communication practices in Chinese oncology contexts, summarising best practices while identifying gaps in knowledge. The chapter also seeks to uncover how clinicians, particularly those in Chinese context, can navigate these cultural complexities to provide better care, especially when discussing sensitive topics such as prognosis and advanced care planning. In doing so, it aims to offer some insights into

J. Pun (✉)
Department of English, The Chinese University of Hong Kong, Hong Kong SAR, China
e-mail: jackpun@cuhk.edu.hk

J. Pun (ed.), *Teaching and Learning Oncology Communication*,
https://doi.org/10.1007/978-981-96-9474-7_2

how oncology communication can be improved in Chinese context, while proposing areas for future research.

Importance of Oncology Communication in the Chinese Cultural Context

To highlight key differences between Western and Chinese communication practices in oncology settings, Table 2.1 below provides a comparative summary that contextualizes how cultural norms influence clinical interactions across these two paradigms. In the Chinese cultural context, communication between clinicians and patients is influenced by high-context communication norms (Zhu, 2019). In contrast to Western low-context cultures, where communication tends to be more explicit and direct, Chinese patients often communicate more indirectly. This means that clinicians should always be sensitive to unspoken cues and subtle expressions, as patients may avoid openly discussing sensitive issues, particularly in cases of terminal illness (Pun et al., 2018). For instance, in the Chinese context, family members and caregivers may prefer to discuss treatment plans without the presence of an elderly cancer patient (Lin et al., 2019; Pun et al., 2021). This family-centred communication style can present challenges in the oncology setting, where transparent and clear discussions are crucial for treatment planning and patient care (Pun et al., 2020).

Family-centred decision-making is a core feature of Chinese culture, which contrasts with the Western emphasis on individual autonomy in doctor-patient communication (Pun et al., 2021). In Chinese families, particularly in serious medical contexts like delivering bad news to patients or discussing treatment options, the family often assumes a central role in making decisions on behalf of the patient (Pun et al., 2023). Family members may act as intermediaries, taking a critical role in controlling the flow of information and decision between the clinician and the patient. This can create complexities in communication, as it may limit the patient's direct involvement in decisions about their own treatments (Xu et al., 2006). The family's desire to shield the patient from potentially distressing information, such as a terminal diagnosis, can further obstruct open communication (Hahne et al., 2020).

Another significant cultural factor is the taboo surrounding death in Chinese society. Discussing death or terminal illness is often avoided, as it is believed to bring bad luck or negatively impact the patient's morale (Dong et al., 2016). Consequently, Chinese clinicians may hesitate to broach topics such as prognosis or end-of-life care, which can lead to inadequate communication around crucial matters like Advanced Care Planning (ACP) (Pun, 2022). Families often play a pivotal role in deciding how much information the patient should receive, with some families preferring to keep the patient in the dark about the severity of their illness, which can create ethical dilemmas for clinicians (Cheng et al., 2019; Mok et al., 2003). This dynamic of hierarchical relationships often intersects with deeply rooted cultural beliefs, such as the taboo surrounding death in Chinese society.

Table 2.1 Western vs. Chinese oncology communication practices

Aspect	Western practices	Chinese practices
Communication style	Low-context, direct, explicit	High-context, indirect, implicit
Truth-telling norms	Emphasis on full disclosure to the patient	Disclosure often filtered or withheld by family to protect the patient
Decision-making Model	Patient autonomy prioritized; individual makes decisions	Family-centred; family members often act as gatekeepers or surrogate decision-makers
Role of family	Family involvement only if permitted by the patient	Family plays a central, sometimes dominant, role in managing information and care decisions
Attitudes toward Death	Open discussion of death and end-of-life planning encouraged	Death is a taboo subject; discussions avoided to preserve hope or avoid "bad luck"
Preferred communication models	Shared decision-making frameworks (e.g., SPIKES, patient-centred care models)	Adapted models such as ARCHES or culturally contextualized SPIKES to accommodate family roles and indirect language
Language use and literacy	Predominantly monolingual, with emphasis on health literacy	Multilingual contexts (Cantonese, Mandarin, English) requiring translanguaging and attention to cultural phrasing
Integration of TCM	Limited or no integration; emphasis on evidence-based biomedical treatments	Co-existence of TCM and Western medicine; patients may alternate or combine treatments, requiring respectful dialogue
Hierarchy in Doctor-patient relationship	Flattened hierarchy; patients often feel comfortable questioning doctors	Steep hierarchy; doctors seen as authority figures, patients often defer without challenge
Ethical orientation	Emphasis on informed consent, autonomy, and individual rights	Emphasis on family harmony, relational autonomy, and collective decision-making

Confucian values also contribute to the hierarchical nature of healthcare relationships in Chinese context, where clinicians are often seen as authoritative figures, and patients may feel less empowered to question or challenge medical advice (Deng et al., 2024; Wong & Pang, 2000; Pun et al., 2020). For instance, some Chinese cancer patients prefer that doctors make the decision about their treatment plans at an early stage, after being presented with various treatment options. This paternalistic approach to care results in an asymmetrical doctor-patient relationship, where communication can be one-sided, with the clinician providing information and the patient passively receiving it (Zhou et al., 2017). While patient-centred care has gained prominence globally, its application in the Chinese context can take into account these cultural nuances. This is highlighted by Pun et al. (2018)'s review that clinicians in the Chinese context should move away from reliance on Western-based communication models, by taking local culture into account when understanding and interpreting medical interactions. For an example, doctors in Chinese context perhaps should involve the family in healthcare decisions and respect their role, which means patient-centered care must be adapted to fit these cultural expectations instead of using only Western methods (See more Pun, 2023). Although there is growing recognition of the need for greater patient involvement, long standing traditions of deference to authority and family involvement continue to shape the dynamics of doctor-patient communication (Banerjee & Sanyal, 2012; Rui, 2015).

In addition to cultural factors, the multilingual and multidisciplinary nature of healthcare in China, particularly in regions like Hong Kong, further complicates oncology communication (Pun, 2021). In many settings, doctor-patient interactions may be through multiple languages—such as Cantonese, Mandarin, and English—making it challenging to ensure that sensitive information is accurately conveyed (Slade et al., 2015). The complexity of these multilingual interactions is compounded by the fact that healthcare professionals often need to switch between languages when discussing medical terminology and everyday communication. For instance, medical records are typically written in English, but verbal communication with patients is often conducted in Cantonese, requiring a form of translanguaging—whereby professionals move fluidly between languages to bridge the gap between medical and everyday language (Pun, 2021). This process, while necessary, introduces risks of miscommunication or incomplete information transfer, particularly when medical terminology has no direct translation in Cantonese or when cultural nuances affect how information is shared (See more from Pun, 2023). Furthermore, the multilingual context can make it difficult for clinicians to ensure patients fully understand critical aspects of their care, particularly regarding sensitive topics such as prognosis or treatment options. Addressing these challenges requires not only language proficiency but also a deep cultural competence that can help clinicians navigate both linguistic and cultural barriers to effective communication in oncology settings.

Moreover, the integration of traditional Chinese medicine (TCM) into cancer care adds another layer of complexity, as communication between professionals from different medical paradigms requires clear and respectful dialogue (Pun & Wong, 2022). The integration of TCM into oncology care presents a unique set of communication challenges and opportunities for clinicians and patients. TCM, deeply rooted in Chinese cultural beliefs and practices, is often viewed by patients as a holistic alternative or complement to Western medical treatments for cancer. This creates a complex landscape in which oncologists and TCM practitioners must navigate differing medical paradigms, while patients may seek to combine or alternate between treatments based on personal or cultural preferences (Pun & Wong, 2022). For many Chinese cancer patients, TCM offers a sense of familiarity and comfort, aligning with cultural values that emphasise balance, harmony, and the body's intrinsic ability to heal itself. Patients often believe that TCM treatments, such as herbal remedies or acupuncture, can strengthen their immune systems, mitigate side effects of chemotherapy, or improve overall well-being (Xu et al., 2006). However, these beliefs can sometimes complicate communication between oncologists and their patients, particularly when there are concerns about the efficacy and safety of TCM in conjunction with conventional cancer treatments. Oncologists in these contexts may find themselves in a delicate position. Many are tasked with respecting their patients' cultural beliefs while ensuring that treatments are evidence-based and medically sound. This dynamic can lead to tension, as oncologists may feel the need to challenge patients' reliance on TCM if it conflicts with conventional treatment protocols, yet must do so in a culturally sensitive manner (Pun & Wong, 2022). On the other hand, TCM practitioners might offer treatments that prioritise improving the patient's quality of life, focusing on long-term health maintenance rather than immediate clinical outcomes, which can diverge from Western medical objectives (Pun & Kong, 2023).

Moreover, effective communication between oncologists and TCM practitioners is crucial in ensuring that patients receive integrated care that avoids potential interactions between TCM and Western medicines (Lam et al., 2009). In the Hong Kong context, fostering better collaboration between TCM practitioners and oncologists is particularly important, as many patients use both treatment approaches, requiring joint efforts to ensure safety and optimize care outcomes (Pun & Wong, 2022). Unfortunately, this collaboration is often underdeveloped due to differences in medical training, language, and treatment philosophies (Pun et al., 2018). Clear, respectful dialogue between these medical systems is essential to providing patients with safe and coordinated care, especially in contexts where patients are navigating both systems (Pun & Kong, 2023). To enhance communication in oncology settings where TCM is integrated, clinicians need to adopt a culturally competent approach. This involves not only understanding the cultural significance of TCM for patients but also actively creating spaces for open dialogue about how TCM and Western treatments can be used safely together. Furthermore, there is a need for more structured collaboration between oncologists and TCM practitioners, ensuring that both parties work towards the shared goal of improving patient outcomes while respecting cultural values (Pun, 2023). In conclusion, the role of TCM in cancer care underscores the importance of culturally sensitive communication strategies. By acknowledging the significance of TCM in the lives of Chinese patients and fostering collaboration between Western and traditional medicine, healthcare providers can better navigate the complexities of oncology care in this unique cultural context.

In addition to addressing the influence of cultural values on oncology communication, this chapter will further explore several key dimensions that impact interactions between clinicians and Chinese cancer patients. Central to these discussions is the role of family in decision-making, where family members often assume a protective role in controlling the flow of information, raising ethical dilemmas for clinicians who must balance patient autonomy with family wishes. Moreover, the challenge of discussing Advanced Care Planning (ACP) in the Chinese context, where death remains a taboo subject, will be examined, along with strategies for engaging patients and families in meaningful discussions about end-of-life care. As healthcare in Hong Kong evolves, the shift towards patient-centered care and its impact on traditional paternalistic approaches will also be considered, offering insights into how patient empowerment is reshaping communication dynamics in oncology. Ethical dilemmas related to truth-telling, confidentiality, and consent further complicate the doctor-patient relationship, particularly in cases of terminal illness. Additionally, this chapter will discuss how spiritual and religious beliefs influence patients' perceptions of illness and death, as well as how technology is being utilized to facilitate better communication in oncology settings. Finally, the importance of clinician training in cultural competence will be highlighted, advocating for comprehensive programs that equip healthcare providers with the necessary skills to navigate these complex cultural and ethical landscapes effectively. Together, these sections aim to provide a holistic understanding of the multifaceted challenges and opportunities in oncology communication with Chinese patients.

1. TheRole of Family inCancer Communication and Decision-Making

In Chinese culture, family plays an integral role in communication and decision-making, particularly when it comes to serious illnesses such as cancer. Unlike in many Western contexts, where patient autonomy is prioritised, Chinese families often assume a central role in managing medical information and decisions on behalf of the patient (Pun et al., 2023). Family members frequently act as intermediaries between the patient and healthcare providers, controlling the flow of information regarding the patient's diagnosis and treatment options. This dynamic is rooted in cultural values that emphasize collective family responsibility and protection of loved ones from distress (Pun et al., 2018).

One of the most significant challenges that arises in this context is the practice of shielding the patient from potentially distressing information, such as the severity of their prognosis or terminal diagnosis. Family members, driven by a desire to protect the patient's emotional well-being, may request that clinicians withhold information about the patient's condition, particularly if it involves terminal cancer or discussions of end-of-life care (Hanson et al., 1997). This practice, while well-intentioned, can create substantial ethical dilemmas for clinicians, who are often caught between respecting the family's wishes and their professional obligation to inform the patient (Cheng et al., 2019). For instance, doctors may struggle with whether to fully disclose the nature of the illness to the patient, as Western medical ethics prioritize patient autonomy and the right to know, while Chinese cultural norms place a higher value on maintaining hope and emotional stability within the family (Mok et al., 2003).

In navigating these delicate situations, healthcare providers must carefully balance the need for transparent communication with respect for the family's cultural values. One approach is to engage in family-centred discussions early in the treatment process, fostering a collaborative decision-making environment where the patient's wishes, as well as the family's concerns, are considered (Michael et al., 2014). This can help mitigate the potential for conflict and ensure that the patient's preferences are honoured without alienating the family. Additionally, clinicians can adopt culturally sensitive communication strategies, such as gradually introducing the patient to difficult topics in a manner that aligns with the family's approach to managing bad news (Pun et al., 2023).

At the same time, it is essential for clinicians to advocate for the patient's autonomy, when possible, especially in situations where the patient's understanding of their condition is necessary for informed decision-making. In some cases, family members may unintentionally undermine the patient's autonomy by withholding critical information, which can prevent the patient from making informed choices about their treatment or end-of-life care (Pun et al., 2023). This highlights the need for healthcare professionals, particularly for those oncologists or allied healthcare professionals in Chinese context, to be skilled in navigating the complex dynamics between patient autonomy and family involvement, offering insights into how these culturally sensitive situations can be managed effectively. Ultimately, while the family's role in cancer communication is shaped by cultural values that emphasize protection and collective responsibility, it is crucial to ensure that the patient's voice is not lost in the process (Epstein et al., 2017). By fostering open dialogue and carefully balancing cultural respect with ethical medical practice, clinicians can help navigate the challenging terrain of family-centred decision-making in cancer care.

2. **Advanced Care Planning (ACP) in theChinese Context**

Advanced Care Planning (ACP) plays a crucial role in ensuring that patients with terminal illnesses receive care aligned with their values and preferences, particularly as they approach the end of life. However, in the Chinese cultural context, engaging in discussions about death, dying, and end-of-life care is often fraught with challenges. Traditional Chinese beliefs, deeply influenced by Confucian and Taoist philosophies, view discussions of death and terminal illness as taboo, associating such conversations with bad luck or the potential to cause emotional distress to the patient and family (Pun, 2022). Consequently, this cultural reluctance creates significant barriers to effective communication around ACP, making it difficult for clinicians to initiate conversations about advance directives, do-not-resuscitate (DNR) orders, and palliative care (Cheng et al., 2019). For example, in Hong Kong, many families may refuse to discuss do-not-resuscitate (DNR) orders with patients, fearing it could diminish their hope and negatively impact their emotional well-being.

One of the primary cultural challenges clinicians face perhaps is the reluctance of both patients and families to openly discuss terminal illness. In many cases, families prefer to avoid informing the patient of their true prognosis, fearing that such knowledge might diminish the patient's hope and accelerate physical and emotional decline (Cheng et al., 2019). This family-centred approach to managing bad news reflects the protective role that families often play in Chinese healthcare settings, where shielding the patient from distress is seen as an act of love and duty (Pun et al., 2021). However, this practice can significantly impede ACP discussions, as it may limit the patient's opportunity to express their preferences for end-of-life care, including their wishes regarding life-sustaining treatments and DNR decisions (Leung et al., 2018).

For oncologists, especially those working with Chinese patients and relatives, navigating these cultural sensitivities perhaps require a delicate balance between respecting the family's wishes and advocating for the patient's right to be informed and involved in decision-making about their own care. One approach is to introduce ACP discussions gradually, allowing families and patients to become more comfortable with the idea over time (Johnson et al., 2016). Clinicians might start by discussing general health preferences and values, slowly transitioning to more specific topics related to end-of-life care as trust is built (Pun et al., 2021). By framing these conversations in terms of ensuring that the patient's dignity and comfort are respected, clinicians can align the goals of ACP with culturally important concepts, such as maintaining family harmony and protecting the patient's well-being (Cheung et al., 2020; Chiang et al., 2021).

Another practical strategy is to involve family members in the ACP discussion from the outset, acknowledging their important role in decision-making. By engaging the family in conversations about the patient's values and preferences, clinicians can help families understand that ACP is not solely about preparing for death, but about ensuring the patient receives care that aligns with their beliefs and desires. This approach can help to alleviate the fear that discussing ACP is tantamount to giving up hope, and instead emphasize that it is a way to honour the patient's wishes (Mok et al., 2003). Additionally, clinicians can provide families with culturally relevant educational resources that explain the purpose and benefits of ACP, helping to demystify the process and reduce anxieties around end-of-life planning (Pun, 2022). For instance, in Hong Kong, clinicians can consider starting ACP discussions by involving both the patient and their family early on, as seen in some hospitals where family meetings are used to address cultural concerns and emphasize that ACP is about respecting the patient's wishes rather than signalling an acceptance of impending death.

Despite the cultural barriers to discussing death and dying, research suggests that when ACP discussions are handled with cultural sensitivity, many Chinese patients and their families are willing to engage in these conversations, particularly if they are framed in a way that respects their values and beliefs (Pun et al., 2023). Clinicians who are equipped with a deep understanding of Chinese cultural attitudes toward death and illness, as well as the communication skills to navigate these complex dynamics, are better positioned to facilitate meaningful ACP discussions that respect both patient autonomy and family involvement (Pun et al., 2020). In conclusion, effective communication about ACP in the Chinese context requires clinicians to approach these conversations with cultural competence, patience, and sensitivity. By recognizing and addressing the cultural reluctance to discuss terminal illness, and by involving both patients and their families in the decision-making process, healthcare providers can ensure that Chinese patients receive end-of-life care that honours their values and preferences.

3. **Patient Empowerment and the Shift Toward Patient-Centred Care**

Healthcare in Hong Kong and China is undergoing a gradual but notable shift toward a more patient-centred care model, reflecting global trends that emphasize patient autonomy, participation, and shared decision-making (Pun, 2023). Traditionally, medical practice in these regions has been characterized by a paternalistic approach, in which doctors and families take primary responsibility for medical decision-making (Tsai, 2001). In this model, patients often defer to the authority of clinicians or allow family members to make critical decisions on their behalf, particularly in the context of serious illnesses such as cancer (Laidsaar-Powell et al., 2016). However, with increasing awareness of patient rights and the growing influence of Western medical practices, there is a movement toward empowering patients to take a more active role in their healthcare (Pun et al., 2018).

The traditional paternalistic approach in Chinese healthcare is deeply rooted in cultural values that prioritize family involvement and respect for authority (Meng et al., 2024). In many cases, patients rely on doctors to make decisions for them, viewing medical professionals as figures of authority whose expertise should not be questioned (Popowicz, 2021). Similarly, families often take on a protective role, managing the flow of information and making decisions on behalf of the patient, especially when dealing with terminal illness (Xu et al., 2006). For instance, in the Chinese context, some doctors may consult with the patient's family first about a diagnosis or treatment plan, sometimes withholding critical information from the patient to protect them from distress, in accordance with family wishes. This approach, while culturally appropriate in many cases such as in Chinese context, can limit the patient's involvement in their own care and reduce opportunities for open communication between the patient and their healthcare team (Pun et al., 2018).

However, the rise of patient-centred care is challenging these traditional practices by promoting greater involvement of patients in decisions about their treatment and care. Patient-centred care is based on the principle that individuals have the right to be fully informed about their health and to participate in decisions that affect their care. This model perhaps shifts the focus from the clinician as the sole decision-maker to a more collaborative approach, where patients are encouraged to express their preferences, ask questions, and engage in discussions about their treatment options (Pun et al., 2020). For instance, some doctors in the Chinese context are beginning to involve patients more directly by encouraging them to ask questions and express their treatment preferences, while still considering the family's input as part of the decision-making process.

In the context of oncology, where decisions about treatment can have profound implications for a patient's quality of life and long-term outcomes, the shift toward patient empowerment is particularly significant. Research has shown that when patients are actively involved in their treatment decisions, they are more likely to be satisfied with their care, adhere to treatment plans, and experience better overall outcomes (Pun et al., 2020; Slade et al., 2015). Moreover, patient-centred communication has been associated with improved psychological well-being, as it allows patients to feel more in control of their health and more confident in their ability to manage the challenges of cancer treatment (Pun et al., 2023).

Despite these benefits, the transition to a patient-centred model in Hong Kong and China is not without challenges. The ingrained cultural values of family-centred decision-making and deference to authority can create tensions between the desire to empower patients and the need to respect family dynamics. For instance, some families may resist efforts to involve the patient in decision-making, preferring to shield them from distressing information or take charge of treatment choices on their behalf (Mok et al., 2003). Clinicians, too, may face difficulties reconciling their professional obligation to promote patient autonomy with the expectations of families who adhere to more traditional approaches to care.

To navigate these challenges, healthcare providers must develop culturally sensitive strategies that respect both the patient's autonomy and the family's role in care. One approach is to adopt a blended model of care that allows for patient empowerment while acknowledging the importance of family involvement. This could involve encouraging open discussions with both the patient and the family, clarifying the patient's preferences, and ensuring that the family's concerns are also addressed. By facilitating a collaborative dialogue, clinicians can help reconcile the patient-centred care model with existing cultural norms, ensuring that both patient autonomy and family harmony are respected (Pun et al., 2023). In addition to fostering open communication, oncologists and related healthcare professionals can support the shift toward patient empowerment by offering patients and families educational resources that explain the importance of patient participation in care (Pun et al., 2021). This can help demystify the concept of patient-centred care, alleviating fears that it undermines the family's role or disrespects traditional values.

In conclusion, the shift toward patient-centred care in Hong Kong and China represents an important evolution in the relationship between patients, families, and healthcare providers (Pun et al., 2018). While cultural norms may present barriers to fully embracing patient empowerment, a blended approach that respects both patient autonomy and family involvement can help bridge the gap between traditional and modern models of care. By fostering open communication, promoting shared decision-making, and providing culturally sensitive support, clinicians can facilitate a smoother transition toward a more patient-centred approach in oncology care.

4. Ethical Dilemmas in Oncology Communication

In the context of oncology, clinicians often face complex ethical dilemmas as they navigate the intersection between medical ethics and cultural norms (Alanazi et al., 2024). Issues such as truth-telling, confidentiality, and patient consent are particularly challenging in the Chinese context, where traditional values may conflict with the ethical principles that underpin Western medical practices (Pun et al., 2020). The cultural emphasis on family-centred decision-making and the taboo surrounding discussions of terminal illness can create significant ethical tensions, especially in cases of advanced or terminal cancer (Pun et al., 2018).

One of the most common ethical dilemmas in oncology communication is related to truth-telling (Buken, 2003; Surbone, 2006). In Western medical ethics, truth-telling is seen as essential to respecting patient autonomy and ensuring that patients can make informed decisions about their treatment. However, in many Chinese families, there is a strong cultural belief that protecting the patient from distressing news is an act of compassion (Pun, 2023; Pun et al., 2023). As a result, family members may ask clinicians not to disclose the full extent of a cancer diagnosis or prognosis to the patient, believing that such knowledge could cause emotional harm, loss of hope, or hasten the patient's physical decline (Cheng et al., 2019). This presents a dilemma for clinicians, who must balance their ethical duty to provide the patient with truthful information with the family's desire to shield the patient from distress.

Confidentiality also becomes a complex issue in this context. In many Western healthcare systems, confidentiality is paramount, with information about a patient's diagnosis and treatment being disclosed only to the patient, unless they provide explicit consent to share it with others (Crico et al., 2022). However, in Chinese families, it is not uncommon for family members to take control of communication with healthcare providers, making decisions on behalf of the patient and sometimes withholding critical information from them (Pun et al., 2023). This raises questions about whose wishes should take precedence—the patient's or the family's—especially when the patient may not be fully informed about their condition. Clinicians may feel pressured to respect the family's wishes for non-disclosure, even when doing so could compromise the patient's ability to make informed decisions about their care (Xu et al., 2006).

Another key ethical issue in oncology communication is patient consent. In Western medicine, informed consent is a cornerstone of ethical practice, requiring that patients be fully informed about the risks, benefits, and alternatives to any proposed treatment before they agree to it (Brown et al., 2011). In the Chinese context, however, the concept of informed consent can be complicated by the involvement of family members in the decision-making process (Pun et al., 2023). In some cases, families may make decisions on the patient's behalf without consulting them, believing that they are acting in the patient's best interests. This paternalistic approach can undermine the patient's autonomy and raise ethical concerns about whether the patient has genuinely consented to their treatment (Mok et al., 2003).

The tension between ethical obligations to inform the patient and cultural imperatives to protect them from distress creates significant challenges for healthcare providers (Rocque & Leanza, 2015). For example, in Chinese culture, healthcare providers may struggle with whether to fully disclose a terminal cancer diagnosis to a patient, as family members might request withholding this information to prevent emotional distress, creating a conflict between medical ethics and cultural expectations. On one hand, clinicians are bound by ethical guidelines that emphasize patient autonomy, transparency, and the right to make informed choices about one's health. On the other hand, they must navigate deeply ingrained cultural values that prioritize family harmony and the emotional well-being of the patient (Parascandola et al., 2002). This can be particularly difficult when dealing with terminal cancer cases, where the stakes are high, and families may be especially reluctant to confront the reality of the patient's condition.

To address these ethical dilemmas, healthcare providers can adopt a culturally sensitive approach to oncology communication (Pun et al., 2018). One potential strategy is to engage the family in discussions about the patient's preferences for receiving information and making decisions (Pun et al., 2023). By framing the conversation in terms of honouring the patient's values and wishes, clinicians can help families understand that truth-telling and patient involvement are not about causing distress, but about ensuring that the patient's dignity and autonomy are respected (Pun et al., 2023). Additionally, clinicians can use gradual disclosure techniques, where sensitive information is introduced incrementally, giving both the patient and the family time to process the news and discuss it together. In conclusion, the ethical dilemmas surrounding truth-telling, confidentiality, and consent in oncology communication are particularly challenging in the Chinese cultural context, where family dynamics and cultural norms often conflict with Western medical ethics. By employing culturally sensitive communication strategies, healthcare providers can navigate these ethical complexities while respecting both the patient's autonomy and the family's protective instincts.

5. The Impact of Religion and Spiritual Beliefs on Cancer Communication

In Chinese culture, religious and spiritual beliefs play a significant role in shaping attitudes toward illness, death, and the afterlife (Yick & Gupta, 2002). These beliefs are deeply intertwined with cancer communication, particularly when it comes to discussing sensitive topics like palliative care, end-of-life decisions, and the concept of a 'good death' (Pun et al., 2020). Understanding the religious and spiritual dimensions of Chinese culture is essential for clinicians seeking to provide compassionate and culturally appropriate care to cancer patients and their families.

At the heart of Chinese cultural practices related to death and illness are philosophical and spiritual traditions such as Confucianism, Buddhism, and Taoism, each of which offers unique perspectives on life, suffering, and the afterlife (Pun et al., 2018). Confucianism, for example, emphasizes the importance of family harmony, filial piety, and respect for one's ancestors (Meng et al., 2024). These values often manifest in cancer communication as a reluctance to openly discuss death or terminal illness, driven by the belief that such conversations could disrupt familial harmony or bring bad luck (Xu et al., 2006). As a result, family members may avoid talking about the patient's prognosis or delay conversations about palliative care and end-of-life decisions, prioritizing the preservation of hope over direct communication.

Buddhist and Taoist beliefs also contribute to how Chinese patients and their families approach illness and death. In Buddhism, suffering is viewed as a natural part of life, and death is seen as a transition to the next life, where one's karma influences the nature of their rebirth (Dillard et al., 2014). For some cancer patients, these beliefs can provide comfort and a sense of peace, particularly in palliative care settings, where spiritual practices such as meditation or chanting may help them cope with pain and anxiety. Taoism, with its emphasis on balance and harmony with the natural order, encourages acceptance of life's cycles, including death (Mok et al., 2003). Patients who hold Taoist beliefs may be more inclined to focus on holistic approaches to care, incorporating Traditional Chinese Medicine (TCM) and other spiritual practices to maintain balance in the body and mind, even as they face terminal illness (Xu et al., 2006).

The concept of a 'good death' is central to Chinese beliefs about dying (Hou et al., 2022). In many Chinese families, a 'good death' is one that occurs peacefully, with the patient surrounded by family and in a state of emotional and spiritual readiness (Liang et al., 2024). This belief is closely tied to ancestor worship, where honouring one's ancestors is a vital part of family life. Ensuring that a family member experiences a 'good death' is seen as a way of fulfilling one's duty to their ancestors and ensuring that their spirit is at peace (Pun et al., 2023). In this context, communication about palliative care and end-of-life decisions should be handled with great sensitivity, as families may wish to control how the patient's final moments are managed, seeking to fulfil their cultural and religious obligations while also minimizing distress for the patient (Pun et al., 2023).

For clinicians, understanding the spiritual and religious beliefs that influence Chinese patients' views on illness and death is essential for effective cancer communication (Dong et al., 2016). Patients who hold strong spiritual beliefs may be more likely to seek comfort in religious practices or may prioritize spiritual well-being over aggressive medical treatments as they near the end of life (Lo et al., 2002). Clinicians must be prepared to engage in conversations about how spiritual beliefs shape the patient's understanding of their illness and their preferences for care. For instance, a patient who believes in karma or reincarnation may approach decisions about life-prolonging treatments differently than a patient who does not hold such beliefs. Spirituality also plays an important role in patient coping mechanisms. Many cancer patients find solace in spiritual practices, which can provide them with a sense of control and peace during a time of great uncertainty (Halstead & Hull, 2001). Practices such as prayer, meditation, or participation in religious rituals can offer patients emotional support, helping them manage the psychological and existential aspects of their illness. For some patients, spirituality becomes a key factor in decision-making, influencing whether they choose to pursue aggressive treatments or focus on palliative care options that prioritize comfort and quality of life (Pun & Wong, 2022). In conclusion, the intersection of religion, spirituality, and cancer communication in Chinese culture is complex and deeply significant. By understanding how religious beliefs influence patients' attitudes toward death, palliative care, and the concept of a 'good death', healthcare providers can offer more empathetic and culturally sensitive support. Clinicians who engage with patients' spiritual needs are better equipped to facilitate meaningful conversations about end-of-life care, ensuring that patients receive care that aligns with their cultural and spiritual values.

6. **Training Programs for Clinicians on Cultural Competence in Oncology**

Cultural competence is essential for clinicians working in oncology, particularly in contexts where cultural values deeply influence communication about illness, prognosis, and end-of-life care (Cain et al., 2018). Targeted training programmes that address cultural sensitivity are crucial for helping healthcare professionals navigate the unique challenges of oncology communication, especially when dealing with diverse patient populations (Wittenberg et al., 2019). For instance, one effective training program for teaching oncology communication could include role-playing scenarios that simulate conversations with patients from diverse cultural backgrounds, allowing clinicians to practice and develop their cultural competence in real-life contexts. Training in cultural competence can be enhanced through a variety of methods, each designed to provide clinicians with practical skills and insights. Simulation exercises are one such method, offering healthcare professionals the opportunity to practise difficult conversations with actors or through virtual scenarios that reflect real-life clinical challenges (Pilnick et al., 2018). These simulations can include discussions about prognosis, treatment options, and end-of-life care, allowing clinicians to rehearse how to communicate sensitively while considering the patient's cultural background.

Role-playing is another effective method that can be used in training programs to help clinicians build empathy and improve their communication strategies (Baile & Blatner, 2014). By adopting the roles of both patient and clinician, participants can gain a deeper understanding of the emotional and cultural complexities that arise during oncology consultations (Butow et al., 2012). For example, clinicians might practise scenarios where they must discuss treatment plans with a patient whose family prefers to shield them from the full extent of their diagnosis—a common situation in cultures that emphasise family-centred decision-making. In addition to role-playing and simulations, cultural immersion programmes provide clinicians with the opportunity to directly engage with the cultural contexts they will encounter in their practice (Liu & Li, 2023). These programmes could include field visits, patient interviews, or even collaborations with cultural experts to deepen understanding of specific cultural norms around illness and death. For instance, in Chinese contexts, where discussing death is often considered taboo, clinicians can learn strategies to approach these conversations with respect for cultural beliefs while ensuring that patients are informed and involved in decisions about their care. Ultimately, these training programmes should aim to equip healthcare professionals with the skills necessary to navigate culturally sensitive conversations, such as those about patient autonomy, end-of-life care, and advanced care planning (Pun, 2023). By fostering cultural competence, clinicians can provide care that is not only medically sound but also aligned with their patients' cultural values and preferences, thus improving the quality of oncology communication and patient outcomes.

In conclusion, improving oncology communication in the Chinese context requires the development of culturally sensitive communication models that address the unique challenges posed by Chinese cultural norms (Pun et al., 2020). It is insufficient to simply apply Western models of patient-centered care; instead, new frameworks must reflect the central role of the family, the cultural importance of indirect communication, and the widespread reluctance to discuss death (Pun, 2023). These culturally appropriate models will help bridge the communication gap between clinicians and patients, ensuring that interactions are not only effective but also respectful of Chinese cultural values (Pun et al., 2018). Furthermore, there is a pressing need for targeted training programmes that focus on building cultural competence among clinicians. Such training should equip healthcare professionals with the skills to handle sensitive conversations regarding death and prognosis, involve family members in a culturally respectful manner, and manage the hierarchical dynamics that often characterize doctor-patient relationships in Chinese contexts (Pun et al., 2021). By improving cultural competence, clinicians will be better prepared to provide holistic care that meets both the medical needs and cultural expectations of Chinese cancer patients, ultimately fostering better patient outcomes.

Discussion Prompts

1 How do Confucian values and family-centred decision-making influence oncology communication practices in Chinese contexts?
2 What are the communication challenges posed by the cultural taboo of discussing death in Chinese society?
3 In what ways does the integration of Traditional Chinese Medicine (TCM) complicate or enrich oncology communication?
4 How can healthcare professionals balance patient autonomy and family wishes when conveying a terminal diagnosis?
5 What strategies are suggested in the chapter to enhance clinician competence in multicultural and multilingual oncology settings?

Reflection Questions

1 Have you encountered or heard of any situations where cultural beliefs significantly affected medical communication? How would you apply the insights from this chapter in such a context?
2 Reflect on your own cultural norms: how do they influence your views on truth-telling, family roles, and death-related discussions in healthcare?
3 What role should clinicians play in promoting Advance Care Planning (ACP) in culturally sensitive environments?
4 How can you, as a future or current healthcare professional, develop skills to address ethical dilemmas like informed consent and confidentiality when family involvement is high?
5 Which communication models or teaching approaches (e.g., role-play, simulation, cultural immersion) discussed in the chapter do you find most promising for enhancing cultural competence?

References

Alanazi, M. A., Shaban, M. M., Ramadan, O. M. E., Zaky, M. E., Mohammed, H. H., Amer, F. G. M., & Shaban, M. (2024). Navigating end-of-life decision-making in nursing: A systematic review of ethical challenges and palliative care practices. *BMC Nursing, 23*(1), 467.

Baile, W. F., & Blatner, A. (2014). Teaching communication skills: Using action methods to enhance role-play in problem-based learning. *Simulation in Healthcare, 9*(4), 220–227.
Banerjee, A., & Sanyal, D. (2012). Dynamics of doctor–patient relationship: A cross-sectional study on concordance, trust, and patient enablement. *Journal of Family and Community Medicine, 19*(1), 12–19.
Brown, R., Bylund, C. L., Siminoff, L. A., & Slovin, S. F. (2011). Seeking informed consent to Phase I cancer clinical trials: Identifying oncologists' communication strategies. *Psycho-Oncology, 20*(4), 361–368.
Buken, N. O. (2003). Truth-telling information and communication with cancer patients in Turkey. *Journal of the International Society for the History of Islamic Medicine, 2*(4), 31–36.
Butow, P. N., Lobb, E., Jefford, M., Goldstein, D., Eisenbruch, M., Girgis, A., King, M., Sze, M., Aldridge, L., & Schofield, P. (2012). A bridge between cultures: interpreters' perspectives of consultations with migrant oncology patients. *Supportive Care in Cancer, 20*, 235–244.
Cain, C. L., Surbone, A., Elk, R., & Kagawa-Singer, M. (2018). Culture and palliative care: Preferences, communication, meaning, and mutual decision making. *Journal of Pain and Symptom Management, 55*(5), 1408–1419.
Chan, E. A., Wong, F., Cheung, M. Y., & Lam, W. (2018). Patients' perceptions of their experiences with nurse-patient communication in oncology settings: A focused ethnographic study. *PLoS ONE, 13*(6), Article e0199183.
Cheng, H. W. B., Shek, P. S. K., Man, C. W., Chan, O. M., Chan, C. H., Lai, K. M., Cheng, S. C., Fung, K. S., Lui, W. K., Lam, C., Ng, Y. K., Wong, W. T., & Wong, C. (2019). Dealing with death taboo: Discussion of do-not-resuscitate directives with Chinese patients with noncancer life-limiting illnesses. *American Journal of Hospice and Palliative Medicine®, 36*(9), 760–766.
Cheung, J. T., Au, D., Ip, A. H., Chan, J., Ng, K., Cheung, L., Yuen, J., Hui, E., Lee, J., Lo, R., & Woo, J. (2020). Barriers to advance care planning: a qualitative study of seriously ill Chinese patients and their families. *BMC Palliative Care, 19*, 1–9.
Chiang, F. M., Wang, Y. W., & Hsieh, J. G. (2021, October). How acculturation influences attitudes about advance care planning and end-of-life care among Chinese living in Taiwan, Hong Kong, Singapore, and Australia. In *Healthcare* (Vol. 9, No. 11, p. 1477). MDPI.
Crico, C., Sanchini, V., Casali, P. G., & Pravettoni, G. (2022). Ethical issues in oncology practice: A qualitative study of stakeholders' experiences and expectations. *BMC Medical Ethics, 23*(1), 67.
Deng, T., Tang, J., Li, J., & He, X. (2024). Exploring the role of traditional Chinese values in shaping health beliefs and decision-making process. *American Journal of Health Behavior, 48*(3), 1–11.
Dillard, S. J., Dutta, M., & Sun, W. S. (2014). Culture-centered engagement with delivery of health services: Co-constructing meanings of health in the Tzu Chi foundation through Buddhist philosophy. *Health Communication, 29*(2), 147–156.
Dong, F., Zheng, R., Chen, X., Wang, Y., Zhou, H., & Sun, R. (2016). Caring for dying cancer patients in the Chinese cultural context: A qualitative study from the perspectives of physicians and nurses. *European Journal of Oncology Nursing, 21*, 189–196.
Epstein, R. M., Duberstein, P. R., Fenton, J. J., Fiscella, K., Hoerger, M., Tancredi, D. J., Xing, G., Gramling, R., Mohile, S., Franks, P., Kaesberg, P., Plumb, S., Cipri, C. S., Street, R. L., Shields, C. G., Back, A. L., Butow, P., Walczak, A., Tattersall, M., ...Kravitz, R. L. (2017). Effect of a patient-centered communication intervention on oncologist-patient communication, quality of life, and health care utilization in advanced cancer: The VOICE randomized clinical trial. *JAMA Oncology, 3*(1), 92–100.
Johnson, S., Butow, P., Kerridge, I., & Tattersall, M. (2016). Advance care planning for cancer patients: A systematic review of perceptions and experiences of patients, families, and healthcare providers. *Psycho-Oncology, 25*(4), 362–386.
Fu, C., & Glasdam, S. (2022). The 'good death'in Mainland China-a scoping review. *International Journal of Nursing Studies Advances, 4*, Article 100069.

Hahne, J., Liang, T., Khoshnood, K., Wang, X., & Li, X. (2020). Breaking bad news about cancer in China: Concerns and conflicts faced by doctors deciding whether to inform patients. *Patient Education and Counseling, 103*(2), 286–291.

Halstead, M. T., & Hull, M. (2001). Struggling with paradoxes: The process of spiritual development in women with cancer. In *Oncology Nursing Forum* (Vol. 28, No. 10).

Hanson, L. C., Danis, M., & Garrett, J. (1997). What is wrong with end-of-life care? Opinions of bereaved family members. *Journal of the American Geriatrics Society, 45*(11), 1339–1344.

Hou, X., Lu, Y., Yang, H., Guo, R., Wang, Y., Wen, L., Zhabg, Y., & Sun, H. (2022). Preferences for a good death: A cross-sectional survey in advanced cancer patients. *BMJ Supportive & Palliative Care, 12*(e4), e570-e577.

Lam, Y. C., Cheng, C. W., Peng, H., Law, C. K., Huang, X., & Bian, Z. (2009). Cancer patients' attitudes towards Chinese medicine: A Hong Kong survey. *Chinese Medicine, 4*, 1–8.

Leung, C. C., Pun, J., Lock, G., Slade, D., Gomersall, C. D., Wong, W. T., & Joynt, G. M. (2018). Exploring the scope of communication content of mechanically ventilated patients. *Journal of Critical Care, 44*, 136–141.

Laidsaar-Powell, R., Butow, P., Bu, S., Charles, C., Gafni, A., Fisher, A., & Juraskova, I. (2016). Family involvement in cancer treatment decision-making: A qualitative study of patient, family, and clinician attitudes and experiences. *Patient Education and Counseling, 99*(7), 1146–1155.

Liang, H. J., Xiong, Q., Lin, P. C., Tsai, J. H., & Preston, N. (2024). 'A good ending but not the end': Exploring family preparations surrounding a relative's death and the Afterlife–A qualitative study. *Palliative Medicine*, 02692163241280016.

Lin, C. P., Evans, C. J., Koffman, J., Sheu, S. J., Hsu, S. H., & Harding, R. (2019). What influences patients' decisions regarding palliative care in advance care planning discussions? Perspectives from a qualitative study conducted with advanced cancer patients, families and healthcare professionals. *Palliative Medicine, 33*(10), 1299–1309.

Liu, J., & Li, S. (2023). An ethnographic investigation of medical students' cultural competence development in clinical placements. *Advances in Health Sciences Education, 28*(3), 705–739.

Lo, B., Ruston, D., Kates, L. W., Arnold, R. M., Cohen, C. B., Faber-Langendoen, K., Pantilat, S. Z., Puchalski, C. M., Quill, T. R., Rabow, M. W., Schreiber, S., Sulmasy, D. P., Tulsky, J. A., & Tulsky, J. A. (2002). Discussing religious and spiritual issues at the end of life: A practical guide for physicians. *Jama, 287*(6), 749–754.

Meng, M., Li, X., Zhao, J., & Hao, Y. (2024). When western concept meets eastern culture: Exploring the impact of Confucianism on shared decision-making in China. *Asia-Pacific Journal of Oncology Nursing*, 100586.

Michael, N., O'Callaghan, C., Baird, A., Hiscock, N., & Clayton, J. (2014). Cancer caregivers advocate a patient-and family-centered approach to advance care planning. *Journal of Pain and Symptom Management, 47*(6), 1064–1077.

Mok, E., Chan, F., Chan, V., & Yeung, E. (2003). Family experience caring for terminally ill patients with cancer in Hong Kong. *Cancer Nursing, 26*(4), 267–275.

Parascandola, M., Hawkins, J. S., & Danis, M. (2002). Patient autonomy and the challenge of clinical uncertainty. *Kennedy Institute of Ethics Journal, 12*(3), 245–264.

Pilnick, A., Trusson, D., Beeke, S., O'Brien, R., Goldberg, S., & Harwood, R. H. (2018). Using conversation analysis to inform role play and simulated interaction in communications skills training for healthcare professionals: Identifying avenues for further development through a scoping review. *BMC Medical Education, 18*, 1–10.

Popowicz, D. M. (2021). " Doctor Knows Best": On the epistemic authority of the medical practitioner. *Philosophy of Medicine*, 2(2).

Pun, J. (2021). Clinical handover in a bilingual setting: Interpretative phenomenological analysis to exploring translanguaging practices for effective communication among hospital staff. *British Medical Journal Open*. https://doi.org/10.1136/bmjopen-2020-046494

Pun, J. (2022). Communication about advance directives and advance care planning in the East Asian context: A systematic review. *Oncology Nursing Forum*. https://doi.org/10.1188/22.ONF.58-70

Pun, J. (2023). *The role of language in Eastern and Western health communication.* Routledge.

Pun, J., & Kong, B. C. K. (2023). An exploratory study of communication training for Chinese medicine practitioners in Hong Kong to integrate patients' conventional medical history. *BMC Complementary Medicine and Therapies, 23*(1).

Pun, J., & Wong, W. (2022). Navigating communication between conventional medicine and traditional Chinese medicine: A case study of patients with cancer in Hong Kong. *Supportive Care in Cancer*. https://doi.org/10.1007/s00520-022-06986-8

Pun, J. K., Chan, E. A., Wang, S., & Slade, D. (2018). Health professional-patient communication practices in East Asia: An integrative review of an emerging field of research and practice in Hong Kong, South Korea, Japan, Taiwan, and Mainland China. *Patient Education and Counseling, 101*(7), 1193–1206.

Pun, J., Chow, J. C. H., Fok, L., & Cheung, K. M. (2023). The role of patients' family members in end-of-life communication: An integrative review. *BMJ Open, 32*(2).

Pun, J., Cheung, K. M., & Chow, C. H. J. (2021). A systematic review of teaching end of life communication: The priorities, the challenges and the scope. *BMJ Supportive & Palliative Care*. https://doi.org/10.1136/bmjspcare-2020-002725

Pun, J. C., Cheung, K. M., Chow, C. H. J., & Chan, W. L. (2020). Chinese perspective on end-of-life communication: A systematic review. *BMJ Supportive & Palliative Care*. https://doi.org/10.1136/bmjspcare-2019-002166

Rocque, R., & Leanza, Y. (2015). A systematic review of patients' experiences in communicating with primary care physicians: Intercultural encounters and a balance between vulnerability and integrity. *PLoS ONE, 10*(10), Article e0139577.

Rui, D. (2015). A family-oriented decision-making model for human research in mainland China. *Journal of Medicine and Philosophy, 40*(4), 400–417.

Slade, D., Chandler, E., Pun, J., Lam, M., Matthiessen, C. M. I. M., Williams, G., Espindola, E., Veloso, F., Tsui, K. L., Tang, S., & Tang, K. S. (2015). Effective healthcare worker-patient communication in Hong Kong accident & emergency departments. *Hong Kong Journal of Emergency Medicine, 22*(2), 69–83. https://doi.org/10.1177/102490791502200201

Surbone, A. (2006). Telling the truth to patients with cancer: What is the truth? *The Lancet Oncology, 7*(11), 944–950.

Tay, K., Lee, R. J. Y., Sim, S. W., Menon, S., Kanesvaran, R., & Krishna, L. K. R. (2017). Cultural influences upon advance care planning in a family-centric society. *Palliative & Supportive Care, 15*(6), 665–674.

Tsai, D. F. C. (2001). How should doctors approach patients? A Confucian reflection on personhood. *Journal of Medical Ethics, 27*(1), 44–50.

Wang, L., Geng, X., Ji, L., Lu, G., & Lu, Q. (2020). Treatment decision-making, family influences, and cultural influences of Chinese breast cancer survivors: A qualitative study using an expressive writing method. *Supportive Care in Cancer, 28*, 3259–3266.

Wittenberg, E., Goldsmith, J., Buller, H., Ragan, S. L., & Ferrell, B. (2019). Communication training: Needs among oncology nurses across the cancer continuum. *Clinical Journal of Oncology Nursing, 23*(1).

Wong, T. K., & Pang, S. M. (2000). Holism and caring: Nursing in the Chinese health care culture. *Holistic Nursing Practice, 15*(1), 12–21.

Xu, W., Towers, A. D., Li, P., & Collet, J. P. (2006). Traditional Chinese medicine in cancer care: Perspectives and experiences of patients and professionals in China. *European Journal of Cancer Care, 15*(4), 397–403.

Yick, A. G., & Gupta, R. (2002). Chinese cultural dimensions of death, dying, and bereavement: Focus group findings. *Journal of Cultural Diversity, 9*(2), 32.

Zhou, M., Zhao, L., Campy, K. S., & Wang, S. (2017). Changing of China's health policy and Doctor-Patient relationship: 1949–2016. *Health Policy and Technology, 6*(3), 358–367.

Zhu, H. (2019). *Exploring intercultural communication*: Language in Action. Routledge

Chapter 3
Being an Oncologist in the Chinese Context: Doctors' Professional Identity and the Oncology Care Process

Qianwen Joyce Yu

Introduction

According to the International Agency for Research on Cancer, the global cancer burden was estimated to have risen to 20 million new cases and 9.7 million deaths in 2022 (World Health Organization, 2022). With cancer being a leading cause of death, oncology care has attracted much scholarly attention in health communication research. This chapter seeks to contribute to this line of research by analyzing doctors' engagement in oncology care from the angle of professional identity construction. The focus of this chapter is on the communication during the oncology care process in the Chinese context where healthcare professionals interact with patients with oncologic diagnoses. Communication is an area of critical importance in oncology care, for it involves the sharing of information as diverse as cancer-related fatigue, cancer-causing infections, quality of life, physical performances, treatment plans, prognosis, survival, and palliative care (Nyrop et al., 2016). Such information is intended to facilitate patients' informed decision-making about therapeutic schedules. There is thus a crucial need to find effective ways to inform and motivate cancer patients and their family members to be actively engaged in communication from diagnosis through survivorship. The goal of this chapter is to learn about the significance the unique characteristics of oncology care have on doctors. This is of particular relevance to health communication researchers who are concerned with interdisciplinary issues involving language and medicine, and are devoted to integrating the largely subjective human experience with the more abstract biomedical world (Hamilton & Chou, 2014; Harvey & Koteyko, 2013; Yu & Pun, 2023).

Previous scholarship has highlighted the complexity of oncology communication (Lindig et al., 2024; Nyrop et al., 2016), partly due to the often markedly

Q. J. Yu (✉)
School of Foreign Languages, Soochow University, Suzhou, China
e-mail: qianwenyu4-c@my.cityu.edu.hk

J. Pun (ed.), *Teaching and Learning Oncology Communication*,
https://doi.org/10.1007/978-981-96-9474-7_3

different requirements and expectations regarding the aims, preferences, and practices involved in communication among participants (e.g. oncologists, patients, family members). This chapter argues that such complexities are also reflected on the level of doctors' professional identity construction, and consequently, that an analysis of how providers and patients construct and negotiate their roles and identities throughout the communication process will contribute to a better understanding of the complexities of oncology care.

In order to explore the part that the social dimensions of communication played in doctors' delivery of oncology care and construction of professional identities, and in the broader professional circumstances of doctors, this chapter narrowed the focus down to three major issues for the case study: how oncology communication was co-constructed in the medical consultations and in the personal narratives of oncologists; what beliefs and attitudes the participating oncologists had about communication and about oncology care; how such beliefs and attitudes were associated with the way oncology communication is enacted.

The study was conducted with oncologists working in five public hospitals in Hong Kong and mainland China, which provides multidisciplinary specialist services for cancer prevention, diagnosis, treatment and wellness services. The research findings shed lipght on some of the common characteristics in doctor-patient communication in the present-day Chinese context, yet some remarkable differences emerged in the oncology setting. Although the results were based in one particular sociocultural context, it is hoped that they add to our knowledge of the complexities of professional lives of oncologists in other situations, what challenges they may face, and how they can be better supported in their professional work and continuing development.

Overview

The Conceptual Foundations of Identity

To paraphrase Sarangi and Roberts (1999), it is through language that we enact who we are and where we belong; moreover, our social lives are linguistically negotiated through discourse. Joseph (2010) also notes that "our very sense of who we are, where we belong and why, and how we relate to those around us, all have language at their center" (p. 9). On a similar note, Burr (2015) sees identity as constructed out of culturally available discourses through which individuals communicate with others. Drawing on this linguistic perspective of identity, individuals are engaged in identity construction as they share their observations and judgments about things, and as they question, pay a compliment to, and voice their dissatisfaction with others. With regards to professional identity, individuals draw on occupationally-relevant discourse, which incorporate institutionally and, if any, non-institutionally sanctioned ways of discussing and interacting as members of a certain profession (Holmes, 2006). For oncologists, their personal narratives come complete with their affiliations with some and their distancing from others, their acceptance of particular social/professional practices and rejection of others, and their claim to membership in particular social/professional communities and not others, all of which provide important information about their identity construction (Bucholtz & Hall, 2005).

In order to capture the dynamics involved in the discursive construction of identity, this study analyzes identity from a poststructuralist perspective, positing that individuals are subjected to cultural forces and discursive practices (Baxter, 2016). Their identities are, according to Baxter (2016), governed by various subject positions, approved by the community or cultures they are involved in, made available to them through discourses and cultural practices within a specific social context. The poststructuralist paradigm is at odds with the essentialist view of identity as a unique and fixed *essence* at the core of a unified subject. For poststructuralists, individuals draw on linguistic resources to claim negotiate, and renegotiate identities, which, reciprocally, contribute to the production and reproduction of new forms of language. Within the poststructuralist paradigm, the positioning perspective focuses on the conceptual relationship between language and identity as a balance between how discourses position individuals as subjects in competing manners and how individuals make their own and others' behaviors socially determinate (Baxter, 2016). This originates from the linguistically oriented line of scholarly work by social psychologists, who seek to explore the socially constructed dimensions of interactions. Davies and Harré (1990), for example, adopt this paradigm to better understand the psychology of 'personhood', zooming in on the elusive question of 'Who am I?'. Their analysis follows the poststructuralist principles that not only recognize the constitutive force of discourse, but also see individuals as emerging through social interaction. To be specific, individuals' senses of self, conscious and unconscious viewpoints and emotions alike, and understanding of the world are shaped by their relationships with others (Harré & van Langenhove, 1999). Such relationships provide individuals with the flexibility to index their identification with particular subject positions and with ways of being, the ongoing process of which is constructed and reconstructed within certain discourses (Weedon, 1997). The actual scope of subject positions assumed by individuals or allocated by others are inevitably limited to options available in a certain sociocultural context, and is likely to be taken up, accepted, declined, or challenged (Harré & van Langenhove, 1999). In addition, there is often a clash among different subject positions, with subjectivity functioning as a site for negotiation between conflicting yet interrelated discourses (Andrew, 2016). In the case of workplace discourse, therefore, a doctor may assume or be assigned several positions as part of their professional identity, revolving around different workplace settings.

Drawing on the poststructuralist portrayal of experience, with its meaning embodied in language, as being subject to dynamic and possibly competing interpretations, this study views the meaning of clinical work as dependent on how doctors interpret their profession and on the discourses that they have access to. Consequently, the experience of communicating with oncology patients and the construction of professional identity are largely contingent on language use and on the potentially contradictory discourses within a specific culture.

Situated in the poststructuralist paradigm, the positioning perspective of identity is closely associated with the notion that we, as social actors, produce and reproduce ourselves through our lived autobiographies (Davies & Harré, 1990). That is, we tell stories, either to ourselves or to others, about the way we have already lived and the way we plan to live our lives, so as to achieve a certain form of consistency and coherence among several subject positions we assume. In other words, such narrative forms enable us to give meaning to our lived experience and to present ourselves and others in a "drama" where we accept different subject positions. This makes narratives an apt characterization of professional identity, as individuals use narratives to make sense of their professional lives over time and to discuss their experience with others. As Giddens (1991) astutely put it, identity construction can thus be viewed as an ongoing narrative project, where individuals collaboratively produce their life stories when interacting with others. The life-story narrative by necessity touches upon work life, in that it gives meaning to doctors' experience of providing oncology care by identifying and interpreting significant events when managing institutional demands and organizational hierarchies. It is in their professional identity construction that they recognize their professional agency in terms of claiming their own sense of selves as well as of achieving their professional growth amidst the institutional and policy requirements. Such identity construction, as this study argues, emerges from doctors' narratives and is constituted and reconstituted in culturally shared discourses.

Methodology

Phenomenology

In view of the critical role of language in shaping and transforming identities situated in certain sociocultural contexts (Bucholtz & Hall, 2005), a qualitative research design is selected for this study to gather work-related stories, to identify critical moments or incidents that would shed light on the meaning that participants give to their professional life, and to explore the part played by providing oncology care in the construction of professional identity. This study adopts phenomenology as its philosophical stance, which functions as an effective way of understanding the reason why participants consciously interpret their experiences (Giorgi, 1997). Specifically, the phenomenological method zooms in on the intentional relationship between the participants and the meaning of the things they are concerned with and are experiencing (Giorgi, 1997). Identifying commonalities among individuals' experiences may generate useful information regarding consistent characteristics between stories, contributing further to the understanding of the nature of individuals' professional practice and development in oncology care. To accomplish this, this phenomenological study follows a '3 + 1' framework incorporating three dimensions (each symbolizing one particular respect of the tensions within the area of phenomenology) and writing (overlapping and reconciling the three dimensions) (Hopkins et al., 2017).

As with other phenomenological research, this study utilizes this framework as a technique to help reveal the diverging viewpoints concerning the topic in focus, as well as to offer a language that researchers can make use of to elaborate on how they resolve the tensions emerging from data. Instead of being fixed and static, researchers do not remain at some fixed and static point during the study; rather, their position hinges on the research questions and context (Hopkins et al., 2017).

The first dimension starts with the essence or the essential structure of a phenomenon, involving the characteristics that make it what it is and distinguish it from other, possibly comparable, phenomena (Smith et al., 2009). The essence primarily pivots around what is common and what may be applied to most examples within the phenomenon. In the meantime, some phenomenologists shift their attention from the more universal interest of essence to individuals' unique experiences. That is, these studies prioritize the particular—the experience of certain groups of individuals with similar backgrounds—and are primarily concerned with the in-depth understanding of each individual's experience (Smith et al., 2009). Although these two lines of studies seem to occupy opposite extremes in a continuum, the negotiation of the particular and the general are, according to Hopkins et al. (2017), far from an either-or proposition. Instead, a warts-and-all search for the essence is based on a close look at the details of individuals' experience. This is because at the deepest level, we may have something in common with an individual whose personal situation appears to be fundamentally different from our own at face value. To some extent, it is the particulars of the individual that can provide convincing evidence of the important aspects embodied in the general. As Gadamer (1998) points out, researchers' engagement with a different participant's story represents a step forward towards the overall understanding of the phenomenon. It is therefore incumbent upon the researchers to move back and forth between examining each participant's narrative account on its own and the collective knowledge of the phenomenon under study.

The second dimension—reduction versus reflexivity—directly addresses underlying tension within the field of phenomenology by targeting the researchers' attitudes towards data taking shape in individuals' stories (Hopkins et al., 2017). In other words, the interpretation of data is largely influenced by whether researchers introduce taken-for-granted assumptions into the research process. This dimension can be seen as a negotiation of how researchers manage their baggage, which refers to researchers' prior education, experience, and beliefs that may be integrated into the study. To paraphrase Finlay (2008), the dimension of reduction versus reflexivity addresses the question regarding how researchers manage the pre-understandings that inevitably exert an influence in the study. The search for the essence of research participants' self-reported experiences requires researchers to temporarily set pre-understandings aside (Finlay, 2008). The act of putting aside researchers' pre-understandings in data interpretation is commonly referred to as reduction, where the scope of researchers' attention is reduced to the topic in focus. This, as Finlay (2008) astutely puts it, helps researchers establish a direct and immediate relationship with the world while experiencing it in lieu of conceptualizing it. To be specific, this encourages researchers to learn about something new through participants' authentic experience, instead of automatically switching to what they already know. From this perspective, such an approach also represents an attempt to objectify the interpretation of data and to enhance scientific rigor, with researchers positioned as detached observers (Hopkins et al., 2017). On the contrary, some phenomenologists argue that researchers' prior knowledge and assumptions are likely to facilitate their understanding of the phenomenon, and at the core of their argument is the co-constitution of an individual and the world as a whole. By highlighting the inextricable link between human and world, they point out that people are not detached from the world and that they make sense of it as they exist within it. In this sense, a researcher's subjectivity may not be something that needs to be resisted and monitored for the trustworthiness of research; rather, researchers can use their pre-understandings to better interpret participant experiences (Glesne, 2016). Instead of resisting it, researcher subjectivity needs to be managed with reflexivity, which refers to the noting, tracking, questioning, and sharing of how researchers shape and are shaped throughout the research process (Glesne, 2016). In responding to this dichotomy of positions, Finlay (2008) points out that it is necessary for researchers to consider the impact of their pre-understandings to encourage openness in learning about participants' self-narrated experiences. What's more, researchers should address the potential tension between reduction and reflexivity through strategically alternating between putting pre-understandings aside for an open phenomenological attitude, and reflexively documenting what they bring to the research as a foundation for further understanding.

The third tension—description versus interpretation—addresses the research question, that is, why researchers seek to gather participants' narratives. Typically, descriptions involve what the phenomenon is, and how it is experienced (Moustakas, 1994). Starting with Husserl, the focus of phenomenology is less on data interpretation on the part of researcher, but more on the description of participant experiences (Hopkins et al., 2017). However, phenomenologists like Heidegger see it as their aim to interpret participant experiences rather than just describe them, which is grounded on the belief that we as human beings are constantly interpreting what surrounds us. By emphasizing the human tendency to interpret life stories as an effective way of understanding the phenomenon of interest, they argue that the so-called 'right' interpretation are virtually nil and that different interpretations are merely different angles of understanding one particular phenomenon. In resolving this apparent tension, researchers are not entitled to one position or the other, but move back and forth among positions (Finlay, 2008). It is important for them to take full advantage of description in demonstrating how participants experience the phenomenon, contributing further to the goal of understanding the influence of these experiences. The dimension of description versus interpretation encourages the combination of researchers' iterative cycling between participants' life stories, and their reflection on their emerging understandings of the phenomenon. This combination repeats as researchers constantly revise their understandings each time they engage with participants' narrative accounts. It culminates in the shared understanding of the phenomenon between researchers and participants, yet both parties are aware that even this understanding is tentative (Hopkins et al., 2017).

As the fourth dimension of this framework, writing overlays the above-mentioned dimensions and is fundamental to phenomenological studies. Here writing does not refer in particular to the writing up for publication purposes, which is generally considered as separate from carrying out the research. In phenomenological research, writing and research are included as comprising the process (van Manen, 1990), as writing allows for the reflective and interpretive process that can help researchers clarify and crystallize thoughts. After data collection, researchers begin to process, reflect on, and revise what they have observed and what participants have talked about, identifying what remains ambiguous and what requires further challenging, analysis, and reading. Writing during this process aids in researchers' interpretation of their interaction with and observations of participants, consequently contributing to a more comprehensive understanding of the phenomenon of interest (Hopkins et al., 2017).

Participants and Research Context

The study presented in this chapter is part of a larger project on doctors' professional identities in the Chinese context. Recruited through convenience sampling, participants included 12 oncologists varying in terms of ages, years of working experience, and both genders from five public hospitals in Hong Kong and mainland China. Prior to the study, research invitations were sent to 35 oncologists in five different public hospitals. The invitations specify the details of the study plan, including the expected duration of the project (i.e. 6 months) and the descriptions of data collection methods. Given the long-term commitment, only 12 oncologists agreed to participate in this study. Although the small sample size limits the generalizability of the research findings, participants' diverse professional experiences derived from oncology care can shed light on oncologists' professional identity construction in the Chinese context. It is noteworthy that cultural differences may have a marked influence upon medical care, particularly in the way providers communicate with patients and their family members.

Ethical approval was obtained before data collection, and all participants were informed of the nature, aim, and data collection methods of the study. As a qualitative researcher, the author engaged in meaning negotiation and construction with the participating oncologists through listening to their narratives, asking essential questions, and sharing her own reflections and observations during interviews (Lincoln & Guba, 2007). This helps the author build rapport with the participating oncologists, and also gather first-hand information concerning their professional practice and personal reflections in caring for oncology patients, further providing much food for thoughts about the dynamics of their professional identities as oncologists in the Chinese context.

Data Collection Design

Data for the present study include participating oncologists' narrative frames—their reflective accounts of their professional experiences in response to researchers' guided questions (Barkhuizen & Wette, 2008)—and in-depth interviews with each participant. Participating oncologists were first invited to finish a researcher-led narrative frame in English, where they provided an autobiographical account of the reasons behind their career choice, their working environment, their personal and professional gains, and their current feelings of being an oncologist. The narrative frames were later complemented by audio-recorded interviews, where participants were asked to expand on their present perceptions and practices with regards to a series of important tasks that doctors are generally believed to perform, such as responding to medical problems, prescribing medication, negotiating treatment plans, explaining medical procedures to patients, and promoting health education (Frank et al., 2010; Kak et al., 2001; Yu & Pun, 2023). Conducted in English, these one-to-one interviews were semi-structured in nature and followed a tentative guide designed by the researcher in general terms. The purpose was to gather information relevant to participants' working experiences, their beliefs about oncology care, and how they constructed their professional identities. Given the co-constructed nature of interviews, oftentimes participants altered the directions of interviews in unexpected but eventually enriching ways. During each interview, the researcher posed additional questions on an ad hoc basis in order to address or clarify any noteworthy incidents in ethnographic observations at the hospital. This addition of interview questions may help the researcher better understand the organizational constraints within which the participating oncologists were working. Moreover, the researcher attended these participants' medical consultation sessions over the course of 6 months to observe their interaction with patients. During the observations, field notes were recorded in a straightforward format including the duration and events of the consultation sessions, the interaction of the participating oncologists with patients and the accompanying family members, and any activities that might be of possible interest to the present research. This is to demonstrate how oncologists' professional identities were enacted, and what part these identities play in their experience of caring for oncology patients. The concurrent use of these data collection techniques enabled the researcher to explore the connections among them. This echoes with some of recommendations proposed by Robson and McCartan (2016) to reduce researcher bias and to enhance research credibility, including extended involvement with participants, consistent observation of the research setting and participants' behaviors, and triangulation of either data sources or data collection methods.

Data Organization and Analysis

The analysis of qualitative data was carried out in a recursive and iterative manner, with the researcher moving between the data (i.e. narrative frames, semi-structured interviews, on-site observation), the analytical framework (i.e. the '3 + 1' framework), and the research aim for a good understanding of oncologists' professional identity construction. Following Miles et al. (2014)'s suggestions about qualitative data analysis, the researcher first reviewed the data repeatedly to identify the themes concerning how participating oncologists perceived themselves and how they were perceived in delivery of oncology care. This step enables key themes to emerge in relevance to participants' professional identities as oncologists. The themes alongside the chunks of data attached to them (i.e. words, phrases, sentences) were then identified to explore how participating oncologists' professional identities were discursively constructed. Particular attention was paid to the role of the researcher as well as of the working environment for interpreting meaning of a text. This is especially helpful for the researcher as both an insider with rooted knowledge of the situated sociocultural context and as an academic outsider with limited knowledge of the profession (i.e. oncology department). Both positions provided the researcher with the critical distance necessary to analyze the data.

Results

This section provides an analytical account of how participating discursively constructed their professional identity as an oncologist. Two major themes emerged from participating oncologists' stories concerning professional identities and their experiences in interacting with and caring for oncology patients. The description of each theme is followed by detailed discussion and further interpretation. Emergence of themes from coding and supporting quotations are presented in the following sections.

Cross-Disciplinary Cooperation

In delivering oncology care, some doctors underwent a profound "reality shock" during their transition from residency training to their role as an oncologist. This was particularly salient at the beginning of their career. Upon their reintegration into the oncology department, it became evident to them that they had progressed to a distinct juncture in their professional journeys, and the prevailing socio-ecological landscape within the oncology department had transformed markedly, with interprofessional collaboration being a case in point.

> Each discipline has their own sort of standpoint and priorities, so I think sometimes its, and obviously it is very important to understand what you may think is a very simple scenario or sort of in terms of knowledge, may be very too, our disciplines may be sort of obvious, it may not be that obvious to other disciplines, after all as a surgeon or orthopedic doctor, whatever, they may not have been managing patients with medical conditions for some time. I've known it ever since the training program that comprehensive cancer treatment requires cross-disciplinary cooperation. Perhaps such cooperation was a bit like instructions coming from my supervisors when I was a trainee. They asked me to contact, well, the general surgery department. I followed the instructions. No questions asked. Right now, it is something indispensable in my daily work. I am on my own, but at the same time I consult my colleagues from other departments. This is part of a standard protocol and I'm so glad that I learned it in training. Such opportunities of communication are very crucial, um, very fundamental. I think again stepping into the shoes of others, understand what they may or may not be aware, I think this is again very important.

In this quote, a participant juxtaposed his experience as a clinical oncology trainee with his current role as an oncologist, highlighting the value he places on interprofessional dialogue throughout his professional development. For instance, while he regarded cross-disciplinary collaboration as an instruction with "no questions asked" in specialist training, he found such collaboration "indispensable" in the current line of work, which made him feel "so glad". Moreover, whereas he had the privilege of seeking guidance from a mentor during his training, he now operated with a greater degree of autonomy. The contrast he drew between these two professional settings (Bucholtz & Hall, 2005) underscores his developmental journey, which has been marked by challenges in adjusting to his current work milieu with the requisite support. This challenge is underscored by his emphatic use of the term "very" to modify "crucial" and "fundamental", indicating his commitment to effective interprofessional communication.

Despite the fact that oncologists had experiences in communicating with professionals from other disciplines during training, they find it challenging to ensure mutual understanding in situations where information exchanges are at stake and communication can be largely compounded by the various contextual factors. Such situations posed severe challenges to the participating oncologists' self-authored identity as an "oncologist-coordinator' in bridging the divisive gap among disciplines that affect medical care and which manifests itself in the multidisciplinary nature of oncology practice. This is exemplified in the quote below, where one participating oncologist, with more than 10 years of working experience, acknowledged that the coordinator role is one that is essential in various problematic or emergency situations. In these contexts, coordinating procedural protocols and medical knowledge among healthcare providers often emerges as an indirect consequence of the cognitive demands placed upon them. As demonstrated in the following quote, the participant clearly marked his rejection of the identity as "doctors who work alone" as a form of "distinction" (Bucholtz & Hall, 2005). Such a rejection underscored his embrace of the role as an "oncologist-coordinator" and his stance was reaffirmed by his response to a preceding inquiry, which was an "if" conditional clause to assert his professional identity. Consequently, the participant's dual roles in delivering medical care and coordinating efforts established the foundation for his oncologist identity, as corroborated by his concluding statement, "That's what we ought to do as oncologists."

Oncologists, like doctors from other specialties, do not work alone. We rely on collaboration and that necessitates communication. Yet communication is not always easy, especially during emergency situations. In suchcritical and messy moments, communication can be chaotic, and our role is to coordinate and to ensure that information is accurately conveyed to our colleagues. It happens so fast and usually we make use of loop communication. Loop communication means that when we give an order, for example we give certain drug, we will yell it out loud and also address it to a specific person. For example, nurse A, please give this patient drug A, fifty milligram through IV access. Can we effectively treat patients if we fail to coordinate the team? Only by managing to coordinate in these communication-critical scenarios can we better utilize our professional knowledge. That's what we ought to do asoncologists.

Oncologist-Patient Communication

Professional identity is further developed with the responsibilities and authority given to oncologists. Many of these responsibilities confer a sense of competence and trust that are reserved for attending oncologists and are tightly knitted into oncologist-patient communication. The qualitative findings were extracted and categorized into three major sub-themes: bad news delivery, decision making, and end-of-life care. Despite the difference in the content, these sub-themes reflect the culture-specific influences of oncologist-patient communication in the Chinese context.

Bad News Delivery

Bad news delivery is a pivotal yet delicate aspect of oncology communication, as it is difficult for oncologists to imagine themselves in their patients' situation when thinking of the details of the unsettling bad news. During the interviews, almost all participants mentioned communication barriers in terms of breaking bad news. These barriers are, to a certain degree, related to the negative attitudes towards death in the Chinese context. For example, one participant brought to light the culture taboos concerning death:

While I want to have can did and thorough discussions with my patients, it is quite difficult. Most of my patients and their families… They do not want that kind of conversation, you know, about terminaldiagnoses. For them, such bad news means bad luck, and I, as the oncologist, am invoking bad luck. I have to spend more time trying to find common ground, sort of like, paving the way for the disclosure. Communicating the diagnosis is my duty and these cultural taboos seem to challenge my identity.

The cultural pressure to avoid discussions of bad news pushed the participant to shift his attention from discussing terminal diagnoses to finding common understanding about the disease (as seen from "have to"). This distinction between the two aspects of his occupational obligations indicated by the conjunction "while" erected hurdles for his identity development as an oncologist. To be specific, as he was driven to allocate more time for a consensus on an honest discussion about the diagnosis, the authenticity of his oncology identity was contested (Bucholtz & Hall, 2005), which is linguistically indexed through the verb "challenge". Although their oncologist identity may be contested as a result of patients' and their family's resistance to communicating bad news, many participants stressed their personal agency in managing the difficulty of responding to patients' emotional distress in diagnosis disclosure:

For anoncologist, communicating diagnosis is always a challenging and stressful endeavor. This is a daunting task. The stakes are high, as itshapes the course of further treatment and prepares the patient mentally for the battle against cancer. Patients would be upset. That's human nature. We had to offer clear information, show empathy and give them time for processing.

The strong evaluative statements such as "This is a daunting task" and adjectives like "challenging" and "stressful" demonstrated the challenges the participant encountered in conveying information related to the disease. In order to meet the occupational requirements, the participant emphasized the need to "offer clear information, show empathy and give them time for processing", which is part of their professional work. This balance between factual and psychological help was also highlighted in the quote below:

I also know that every time you break bad news, it can be very hard emotionally on the patients and their family members. And so part of my work is also to be very attuned to their emotional reaction, and to take things at their pace rather than my pace. I need to let them know that these feelings are normal and they are not in this alone. They would trust you and this type of therapeutic relationship would be sustainable. Communicating medical information is important, but responding to patients'emotional needs is equally important as well. These two tasks should complement each other.

In this quote, the participant commented that addressing emotional responses and validating patients' feelings are an essential complement to medical treatment. This helps prevent patients from experiencing a sense of abandonment. The participant's professional agency as an oncologist was authenticated and strengthened through the resolute modality (e.g. the use of "need" and "should"). Patients' perspectives, from the participant's point of view, should be taken into account in bad news delivery to establish a trusting and sustainable relationship during the treatment.

In terms of communication strategies for breaking bad news, a patient-centered approach to communication was mentioned and favored by most of the oncologists interviewed. According to Epstein et al. (2005), a patient-centered care approach is primarily concerned with four major domains: the patient's perspective, the psychosocial context, shared understanding, and sharing power and responsibility.

For example, one participant shared her experience of considering patients' perspectives in communicating unsettling news. By allowing patients to "ventilate themselves", the participant was able to embark on bad news delivery in a manner that demonstrates care and empathy:

I think we need to try to bring each party to step in to the shoes of other party and incritical illness it's very difficult. Empathy is required. Because emotions are running very high so you really have to try to let them express themselves first and then give them the space to try to step into the shoes of the other party and that really helps if they're able to first ventilate themselves then they will be able to take in the feeling of the opposing party as well. This helps us build trust.

In engaging in verbal discussions of bad news, participants also utilized various materials as aids to facilitate patients' understanding, often of complex specialist terms and processes. As the following quotes demonstrate, supplementary illustrations, diagrams, and pamphlets were used as facilitators to enhance patients' comprehension:

For verbal communication, usually we will need to use simple words that I have mentioned and drawing diagrams and also sometimes we make use of pamphlets that we prepare or videos. We actually have quite a number of videos, teaching the patient about what to expect when they have a stoma. For example, how they should take care of the stoma and how it would look like, which position it would be at.

If necessary, while in fact it's very commonly, I would use some diagrams, illustrations, and also some models, to explain things and then I think it would be easier when we talk about the bad news.

Notably, for oncologists practicing in the Chinese context, cultural competence and family influence can also greatly affect the discussion of upsetting information with patients. Apart from considering patients' perspectives, participants also point out the role of cultural issues in the establishment of a trusting and collaborative doctor-patient relationship in oncology care. To be specific, approval and support from family can provide reassurance that the patient is treated with dignity and respect. For example, one participant pointed out the importance of acknowledging family members' contribution at the outset of bad news delivery:

We will also have to identify and remove common barriers to acceptance of the bad news—if a family member feels guilty of not taking good care of the patient previously, they will try to do their best by placing demands and asking for more from healthcare team taking care of them and ask for more. Make sure they know that the disease has its own natural course and is usually difficult to be picked up at itsearly stage, try to reassure them they have already been doing what they could.

According to her response, family members feelings of guilt in communicating the diagnosis should be acknowledged and addressed. Although challenging, this process can help lay a solid foundation for further treatment. Findings also suggest that attention to family reactions is closely associated with the establishment of a therapeutic alliance:

Very importantly, make them feel that we treat them on a whole, when we ask for questions, when we explain things. I always explain to them together, so that afterwards they can discuss among themselves. And they would also feel better that the patient is being accompanied by his or her family, and that would make him or her feel much better as well. I don't think it's dispensable. It is part of my job.

Usually patients and family need some time to digest and formulate their questions and their concerns after receiving the bad news. So, usually we will spend more time and talk to them properly about the expectation management, for example. What they would like to know about the diagnosis, how they feel at the moment, etc.

In the above-mentioned quote, participants commented on the necessity of responding to perspectives of both patient and family. Given the family oriented Chinese culture, they suggested exploring the patient's and family's perspective appropriately with a focus on their understanding and expectations associated with biomedical concern and emotional distress.

Decision Making

Participants also highlighted decision making as a crucial aspect of communication within their communities of practice, amidst the myriad of responsibilities they encounter. In Chinese culture, medicine holds a position of high esteem as a profession. Patients place significant reliance on doctors for detailed information concerning their diagnoses. They anticipate that their physicians will offer a comprehensive overview of their diagnosis, along with supplementary details that can facilitate their decision-making concerning treatment plans (Fan et al., 2019). This can be seen from the following quote:

Patients, family, they are relying on me. How can I explain in a way to help them grasp their situation and make decision about the treatment and how to comply to the treatments, so that's a unique set of challenges here.

With shared decision-making being valued in patient-centered care, participants were very much aware of the effects of decision-making and expressed a need to ensure that patients were both informed about and involved in the medical decisions that might affect their lives. For example, one participant mentioned the major drive behind careful management of the decision-making process:

Sometimes client and family have unrealistic expectation of outcomes, so we have to make sure we are on the same page. We can explain using figure and facts, we candisclose prognosis using other's experience so they don't take it personal but they know what's expected. I am doing my job, my job as anoncologist. Now that the doctor-patient relationship is rather strained, understanding patients' and their family's expectations play an important role in medical decision making. If you, if you do that, I mean, it's not just about fulfilling the hospital's requirement, it's for self-protection as well. I cannot afford a law suit.

By foregrounding his identity as an oncologist, the participant emphasized the necessity of eliciting and understanding patients' and their family's expectations in discussing medical decisions, which was not only driven by institutional demands, but also had the potential of protecting oncologists from medical complaints. This viewpoint regarding the effect of expectations was further stressed by another participant:

Its delivery of essential information, adequatefor patient to know what's happening and make decision for further care. Part of being anoncologist is about answering patient's additional concerns, to explain the treatment alternatives, and to identify the challenges our clients' currently facing, including physical, psychological, social circumstances, family related. It's about drawing the real picture and maintaining realistic hope.

From his perspective, it is crucial for oncologists to elucidate the available options, accompanied by a suitable amount of scientific information, in order to provide their patients with a holistic understanding of their medical condition and prognosis, steer them through the decision-making process, and aid them in arriving at a satisfactory choice.

In the process of medical decision making, there is often a power differential between patients and doctors (Wang, 2010). In the Chinese context, doctors often play the authoritative role and patients are more passive. Conventionally, it is anticipated that patients would speak less and listen more, refraining from posing numerous questions, as this could be perceived as questioning the doctor's authority. However, the roles and statuses of both clinicians and patients have undergone continuous transformation over time, resulting in a more balanced relationship today than ever before. Both parties now necessitate mutual reliance to engage in a candid dialogue. For example, one participant highlighted the need for a culturally sensitive and family-oriented approach to communicating with patients, to better address the distinct Chinese conceptions of shared decision-making:

Collusion is common in Chinese culturewe usually explore reason why they want to hide the news from the patients, make surethe family understand. Hiding essential information fromthe patient can make patients more stressed, and reassure them you will do this gently. Family takes important role in decision-making, at least in this department. Be sure to involve close family members. Be sensitive to family dynamics, identify carer stress, identify and invite key-person fordecision making. I try my best to do that as anoncologist working in a Chinese hospital.

In addressing the cultural preference in decision making, the participant emphasized that she would "try her best to" encourage patients and family to provide input and participate actively in decisions. For instance, she argued against the concealment of essential information and endeavored to involving patients and family in choices to the degree that they accepted. In doing so, the participant sought to strike a balance between the institutional requirement for medical care and her self-beliefs as an oncologist working in a Chinese hospital by maintaining a strong cultural orientation in her communication.

Broader Considerations in Oncology Communication: Curative Treatments, Complex Decisions, and Financial Concerns

While this chapter has thus far focused on communication challenges related to end-of-life care and shared decision-making, many oncologists also face intricate communication demands when discussing curative treatment options and associated decisions. These conversations often involve highly technical medical information, managing patient expectations, and navigating socioeconomic concerns that can influence patients' choices.

Participants in this study emphasized that curative treatment plans—such as surgery, chemotherapy, and immunotherapy—often come with complicated risk-benefit profiles. Oncologists must translate this information into accessible language while maintaining realistic hope and minimizing false expectations. Several interviewees reflected on the difficulty of balancing optimism with honesty, particularly when discussing outcomes of novel therapies or the likelihood of remission.

> "Sometimes patients hear about advanced therapies on the internet or from friends. I need to help them distinguish between what's possible and what's appropriate in their case. I have to guide them, especially when they want 'the best treatment,' but they might not fully understand the risks."

In addition to clinical complexity, participants also highlighted the impact of financial pressures on communication. In both Hong Kong and mainland China, affordability remains a sensitive issue in cancer care. Patients and families may struggle to weigh therapeutic benefits against treatment costs, particularly when out-of-pocket expenses are high for advanced drugs or private services.

> "It's always difficult when I know a treatment could help, but it's not subsidized. We try to explain options honestly, but there's always the tension between medical recommendation and financial burden. Families often need time to talk it through."

These dilemmas underscore the importance of framing oncology communication within broader social determinants of health. As seen in the narratives, financial barriers can become part of the decision-making dialogue, where clinicians must provide compassionate support while helping families reach feasible, informed choices.

Recognizing these additional dimensions—curative goals, complex choices, and financial discussions—broadens our understanding of oncologists' communicative roles and further reinforces how professional identity is negotiated at the intersection of medical expertise, emotional labor, and socioeconomic realities.

Discussion

This phenomenological study, informed by a poststructuralist approach, explores how oncologists constructed and reconstructed their professional identities in their medical practice. Cross-disciplinary collaboration with colleagues, and communication with patients and family in the delivery of oncology care can be seen as the key sites for the social constructions of professional identities for the research participants. Communication constitutes an essential locus for enacting institutional roles and relationships and oncologists can play a fundamental role in mediating these relationships and fulfilling work-related objectives. As qualified oncologists maneuver their way through the paradoxical landscape of oncology care, interactions within their communities of practice help brew identity work in the wider sociocultural and professional context.

As the data presented in the preceding section demonstrates, being an oncologist is accomplished interactionally and various providers from different disciplines participate in the diverse processes involved in the construction of professional identities. This is in line with Chan et al. (2018)'s argument that professional identity construction is marked by both a personal and institutional recognition of these individuals displaying knowledge, attitudes and behaviors beyond those expected in medical trainees. With interprofessional collaboration being a crucial component of patient-centered and comprehensive healthcare services (Fox & Reeves, 2014), healthcare organizations across the globe are mandating an interprofessional team-based approach in medical practice (Fox et al., 2021). In teamwork-based oncology care, participants describe themselves and are constructed by others as the one in charge and the coordinator of the team. For example, participants regularly engage in discursive practices of relevance to certain stances indexed for the enactment of power and authority, such as holding routine meetings, and designating responsibilities and assigning tasks. Apart from these practices, the collaborative actions that support multi-vocality further contributes to constructing participants' professional identity as an oncologist.

In addition to the comparatively uncontested ways of doing identity work in cross-disciplinary communication, findings have also shown that participants' professional identity as an oncologist may be challenged in their communication with patients and family. Such challenges are, to a certain degree, associated with dynamic discourse moves that require additional sociocultural knowledge to be understood. As seen in the study, the interdependence on family members and negative attitudes towards bad news remain particularly powerful in medical discourse situated in the Chinese context. Communicating with patients and their family members in oncology care can be stressful and technically demanding for providers (Pun et al., 2020), for it is by necessity influenced by the cultural preference for avoiding disclosure of unfavorable diagnosis (Fan et al., 2019). This presents challenges for participants' provision of emotional support and consequently challenge the authenticity of their professional identity as an oncologist. Also, patients' preferences for a family-driven decision require oncologists to aim for a shared understanding of the medical problem and its treatment with both patients and their family. This means that effective communication here is positively conditioned by an understanding of both parties' perspectives including their concerns, feelings, and expectations. In order to cope with these challenges, participants manage to exercise their agency in adopting a family-oriented approach in communication in balancing professional goals and institutional demands.

Overall, oncologists' identity work is a two-way process: while they seek to form their professional identities through different forms of interaction, their identities were inevitably subjected to sociocultural influences such as a cultural and a familial dimension to the Chinese construct medical communication. As healthcare reform progresses further within the Chinese context (Tang & Guan, 2017), oncologists are poised to confront a growing array of institutional challenges and demands that may diverge from their practice orientations and undermine their autonomy. Consequently, this poses a pivotal yet challenging inquiry: what measures can healthcare institutions adopt to assist oncologists in preserving and enhancing their professional identities? While this may be beyond the scope envisaged for the present study, longitudinal research is needed to provide more insights into the multifaceted and contested nature of oncologists' professional identities in relation to their embedded sociocultural contexts.

Discussion Prompts

1 How does the poststructuralist view of identity help explain the communication practices of oncologists in the Chinese healthcare system?
2 What are the key challenges to professional identity construction for oncologists in cross-disciplinary and family-oriented communication contexts?
3 How do oncologists in this study negotiate their role between institutional demands and patient-centered care, particularly when delivering bad news?
4 What insights does the chapter offer about the importance of reflexivity in qualitative health research, especially when examining professional identities?
5 How does the Chinese cultural context (e.g., attitudes toward death, family involvement) shape oncologist-patient communication differently from Western models?

Reflection Questions

1 Reflect on the dual role of oncologists as both clinicians and coordinators. How might this affect their communication style and professional identity?
2 What strategies could you adopt in your own clinical or academic work to better support identity development among early-career medical professionals?
3 How has this chapter influenced your understanding of the importance of family dynamics in oncology care communication in culturally specific settings?
4 What are your thoughts on the use of narrative methods in exploring professional identity? What are the strengths and limitations of this approach?
5 How might the findings in this chapter help improve interdisciplinary communication and training within your own institution or practice?

References

Andrew, P. (2016). Constructing age identity: The case of Mexican EFL learners. In S. Preece (Ed.), *The Routledge handbook of language and identity* (pp. 337–350). Routledge.

Barkhuizen, G., & Wette, R. (2008). Narrative frames for investigating the experiences of language teachers. *System, 36*(3), 372–387. https://doi.org/10.1016/j.system.2008.02.002

Baxter, J. (2016). Positioning language and identity: Poststructuralist perspectives. In S. Preece (Ed.), *The Routledge handbook of language and identity* (pp. 34–49). Routledge.

Bucholtz, M., & Hall, K. (2005). Identity and interaction: A sociocultural linguistic approach. *Discourse Studies, 7*, 585–614. https://doi.org/10.1177/1461445605054407

Burr, V. (2015). *Social constructionism* (3rd ed.). Routledge.

Chan, M., Pratt, D., Poole, G., & Sidhu, R. (2018). Professional paradox: Identity formation in qualified doctors pursuing further training. *Medical Education, 52*(3), 302–313. https://doi.org/10.1111/medu.13485

Davies, B., & Harré, R. (1990). Positioning: The discursive production of selves. *Journal for the Theory of Social Behaviour, 20*(1), 43–63. https://doi.org/10.1111/j.1468-5914.1990.tb00174.x

Epstein, R., Franks, P., Fiscella, K., Shields, C. G., Meldrum, S. C., Kravitz, R. L., & Duberstein, P. R. (2005). Measuring patient-centered communication in patient-physician consultations: Theoretical and practical issues. *Social Science & Medicine, 61*(7), 1516–1528. https://doi.org/10.1016/j.socscimed.2005.02.001

Fan, Z., Chen, L., Meng, L., Jiang, H., Zhao, Q., Zhang, L., & Fang, C.-K. (2019). Preference of cancer patients and family members regarding delivery of bad news and differences in clinical practice among medical staff. *Supportive Care in Cancer, 27*(2), 583–589. https://doi.org/10.1007/s00520-018-4348-1

Finlay, L. (2008). A dance between the reduction and reflexivity: Explicating the "Phenomenological Psychological Attitude." *Journal of Phenomenological Psychology, 39*, 1–32. https://doi.org/10.1163/156916208X311601

Fox, A., & Reeves, S. (2014). Interprofessional collaborative patient-centred care: A critical exploration of two related discourses. *Journal of Interprofessional Care, 29*(2), 113–118.

Fox, S., Gaboury, I., Chiocchio, F., & Vachon, B. (2021). Communication and interprofessional collaboration in primary care: From ideal to reality in practice. *Health Communication, 36*(2), 125–135.

Frank, J. R., Snell, L. S., Cate, O. T., Holmboe, E. S., Carraccio, C., Swing, S. R., Harris, P., Glasgow, N. J., Campbell, C., Dath, D., Harden, R. M., Iobst, W., Long, D. M., Mungroo, R., Richardson, D. L., Sherbino, J., Silver, I., Taber, S., Talbot, M., & Harris, K. A. (2010). Competency-based medical education: Theory to practice. *Medical Teacher, 32*(8), 638–645. https://doi.org/10.3109/0142159X.2010.501190

Gadamer, H. G. (1998). *Truth and method* (2nd rev. ed. / trans revised by Joel Weinsheimer and Donald G. Marshall. ed.). Continuum.

Giddens, A. (1991). *Modernity and self-identity: Self and society in the late modern age.* Polity Press in association with Blackwell.

Giorgi, A. (1997). The theory, practice, and evaluation of the phenomenological method as a qualitative research procedure. *Journal of Phenomenological Psychology, 28*(2), 235–260. https://doi.org/10.1163/156916297X00103

Glesne, C. (2016). *Becoming qualitative researchers: An introduction* (5th ed.). Pearson.

Hamilton, H. E., & Chou, W. Y. S. (2014). *The Routledge handbook of language and health communication.* Routledge.

Harré, R., & van Langenhove, L. (1999). *Positioning theory: Moral contexts of intentional action.* Blackwell.

Harvey, K., & Koteyko, N. (2013). *Exploring health communication: Language in action.* Routledge.

Holmes, J. (2006). *Gendered talk at work : Constructing gender identity through workplace discourse.* Blackwell.

Hopkins, R. M., Regehr, G., & Pratt, D. D. (2017). A framework for negotiating positionality in phenomenological research. *Medical Teacher, 39*(1), 20–25. https://doi.org/10.1080/0142159X.2017.1245854

Joseph, J. (2010). Identity. In C. Llamas & D. Watt (Eds.), *Language and identities.* Edinburgh University Press.

Kak, N., Burkhalter, B., & Cooper, M. A. (2001). Measuring the competence of healthcare providers. *Operations Research Issue Paper, 2*(1), 1–28.

Lincoln, Y. S., & Guba, E. G. (2007). But is it rigorous? Trustworthiness and authenticity in naturalistic evaluation. *New directions for evaluation,*(114), 15–25. https://doi.org/10.1002/ev.223

Lindig, A., Mannagottera, L., Hahlweg, P., Sigl, H., Klimesch, A., Zeh, S., Kriston, L., & Scholl, I. (2024). Effects of a shared decision-making implementation programme on patient-centred communication in oncology—Secondary analysis of a randomised controlled trial. *Health expectations : an international journal of public participation in health care and health policy, 27*(2), e14030-n/a. https://doi.org/10.1111/hex.14030

Miles, M. B., Huberman, A. M., & Saldana, J. (2014). *Qualitative data analysis: A methods sourcebook* (3rd ed.). SAGE Publications.

Moustakas, C. E. (1994). *Phenomenological research methods.* Sage.

Nyrop, K. A., Deal, A. M., Williams, G. R., Guerard, E. J., Pergolotti, M., & Muss, H. B. (2016). Physical activity communication between oncology providers and patients with early-stage breast, colon, or prostate cancer. *Cancer, 122*(3), 470–476. https://doi.org/10.1002/cncr.29786

Pun, J. K. H., Cheung, K. M., Chow, J. C. H., & Chan, W. L. (2020). Chinese perspective on end-of-life communication: A systematic review. *BMJ Supportive & Palliative Care*, bmjspcare-2019. https://doi.org/10.1136/bmjspcare-2019-002166

Robson, C., & McCartan, K. (2016). *Real world research: A resource for users of social research methods in applied settings.* John Wiley & Sons Ltd.

Sarangi, S., & Roberts, C. (1999). *Talk, work and institutional order: Discourse in medical, mediation and management settings.* Mouton de Gruyter.

Smith, J., Flowers, P., & Larkin, M. (2009). *Interpretative phenomenological analysis: Theory, method and research* (Vol. 6). Sage Publications.

Tang, L., & Guan, M. (2017). Rise of health consumerism in China and its effects on physicians' professional identity and the physician-patient relationship and communication. *Health Communication, 33*(5), 636–642. https://doi.org/10.1080/10410236.2017.1290015

van Manen, M. (1990). *Researching lived experience: Human science for an action sensitive pedagogy* (1 ed.). State University of New York Press.

Wang, Q. (2010). *Doctor-patient communication and patient satisfaction: A cross-cultural comparative study between China and the U.S* [Doctoral Dissertation, Purdue University].

Weedon, C. (1997). *Feminist practice and poststructuralist theory.* Blackwell.

World Health Organization. (2022). *Global cancer observatory: Cancer today.* https://gco.iarc.who.int/media/globocan/factsheets/cancers/39-all-cancers-fact-sheet.pdf

Yu, Q. J., & Pun, J. (2023). Promoting patient engagement in medical informed consent—A qualitative study of Chinese doctors' communication strategies. *Health Communication, 38*(1), 71–79. https://doi.org/10.1080/10410236.2021.1932287

Chapter 4
Language Matters: Breaking Bad News to Chinese Cancer Patients

Kexin Tan

Chapter Summary
This chapter explores the critical task of delivering bad news in oncology, particularly within China's unique cultural landscape. It emphasizes the impact of effective communication on patients' well-being and examines barriers faced by healthcare professionals. Cultural nuances significantly influence how terminal diagnoses are disclosed, with a tension between traditional family views and individual preferences. The SPIKES protocol provides a foundation for delivering bad news, but adaptation to China's context is essential. By mastering linguistic subtleties and fostering cultural competence, healthcare providers can navigate this delicate task with empathy, ensuring patients experience dignity and compassion throughout their cancer journey.

Introduction

The delivery of bad news in healthcare is an important communication skill that bears a significant impact on patients' well-being. Defined as "any information which adversely and seriously affects an individual's view of his or her future" (Buckman, 1992), it is a moment that can define the trajectory of a patient's journey. This holds particularly true in the speciality of oncology, where physicians are often required to discuss life-altering diagnoses and treatment outcomes. Such discussions can be especially difficult due to the potential for cancer diagnoses to result in a host of adverse events, including aggressive treatments that may lead to disfigurement or disability, severe pain, loss of function, and even mortality. These dialogues can be

K. Tan (✉)
Department of English and Communication, The Hong Kong Polytechnic University, Hong Kong, China
e-mail: kexin.tan@connect.polyu.hk

J. Pun (ed.), *Teaching and Learning Oncology Communication*,
https://doi.org/10.1007/978-981-96-9474-7_4

exceedingly stressful and intricate for physicians, necessitating a communication approach tailored specifically to the oncology context—a departure from strategies employed in other bad news scenarios (Parker et al., 2001). Conveying bad news with empathy and understanding is not only a professional obligation, but the foundation of compassionate care. Effective communication can mitigate the distress associated with bad news, helping patients maintain hope amidst challenging circumstances (Buckman, 1996). Conversely, an insensitive delivery can negatively affect patients' perspectives regarding their future (Buckman, 1984).

Cultural differences significantly influence the disclosure of terminal diagnoses to cancer patients worldwide. In the United States, doctors generally favour full disclosure (Novack et al., 1979), but this approach varies widely in many other countries due to cultural perceptions of harm and nonmaleficence. Within Chinese communities, families often resist informing the patient of a dire diagnosis, and doctors in China often communicate with family members instead (Tse & Fok, 2003). Despite this tradition, recent research indicates a growing public desire for transparency, even when the news is unfavourable (Liu et al., 2018). This reveals a stark discrepancy between traditional family views and individual preferences regarding information disclosure, as well as a misalignment between medical practices and patient wishes.

While existing guidelines such as the SPIKES protocol (Setting, Perception, Invitation, Knowledge, Empathy, Strategy) offer a foundation for delivering bad news (Baile et al., 2000; Kaplan, 2010), there is an opportunity for deeper exploration into how these can be thoughtfully tailored to resonate with the Chinese cultural context, where sensitivity to cultural nuances is essential. In Chinese cultural practices, the subtleties of language—from word choice to non-verbal cues—play a pivotal role in communication. These linguistic elements are reflective of underlying values such as collectivism and family solidarity, which guide preferences for a more nuanced and collective approach to decision-making (). It is incumbent upon physicians to master these linguistic subtleties, ensuring that the delivery of bad news is not only respectful but also culturally congruent.

This chapter begins by outlining the objectives of delivering bad news, providing a foundation for understanding its significance. It then examines the barriers to conveying difficult information within China's oncology healthcare system, exploring the cultural factors that underpin these challenges. To address these barriers, the structured SPIKES protocol is introduced and its current application in China is discussed, with an emphasis on the need for culturally-sensitive adaptation.

The chapter aims to equip healthcare professionals with the cultural and linguistic understanding necessary to handle the delicate task of delivering bad news to Chinese cancer patients. It underscores the importance of cultural competence in establishing trust, supporting patient autonomy, and creating a compassionate environment for patients and their families throughout their cancer journey. By integrating ethical communication practices with cultural awareness, the ultimate goal is to provide information while also offering comfort and guidance, ensuring patients experience dignity and empathy.

The Goals of Breaking Bad News

Sweeny et al. (2011) outline six key objectives in the delivery of bad news: (1) ensuring that patients receive clear and comprehensive information about negative outcomes, (2) encouraging patients to follow medical advice, (3) reducing the emotional impact on patients when they receive bad news, (4) enhancing patient contentment with the care provided, (5) fostering patient hope and optimism, balanced with candour and realism, and (6) alleviating the discomfort healthcare professionals may feel due to anticipated patient reactions, their own emotions, or perceived lack of skill. The following analysis of barriers draws upon semi-structured interviews conducted by Dr. Jack Pun in 2021 with six oncologists practicing in China. A thematic analysis of these interviews revealed four primary barriers that complicate the delivery of bad news in the Chinese context. Pseudonyms instead of real names have been used to protect participant anonymity.

Barries of Breaking Bad News in the Chinese Context

Barrier 1: Divergent Perceptions

A recurrent theme was the challenge of managing fundamentally different perspectives between the healthcare team and the patient's family. Participants reported that families often arrived with preconceived expectations about the patient's condition or prognosis, shaped by inconsistent information received from other healthcare providers prior to the oncology consultation. This creates an immediate conflict in perceptions that must be navigated (Dr. A & Dr. B). "It [the differing expectations] is actually quite disturbing because the patient would think that this disease is the end of the world, whereas we actually treat it as a normal encounter day in and day out," as one participant noted (Dr. B). Challenge of bridging the between clinical routines and Dr. C suggested the use of tangible data to manage expectations and to address emotional reactions to treatment outcomes, asserting that "no longer treating doesn't mean neglect".

Additionally, the interviews highlighted that the family unit per se is not monolithic and individual members possess varying capabilities to understand complex medical information. As Dr. D mentioned, different relatives have different comprehension abilities influenced by a combination of factors such as educational background, language proficiency, and even their immediate emotional state. Consequently, a key skill for clinicians is the ability to tailor the disclosure of information accordingly, emphasizing the need for adaptability and empathy from all parties involved in the medical consultation.

Barrier 2: Management of Emotional Reactions

The data indicates that divergent perceptions between doctors and the patient's family are often a surface manifestation of deeper emotional distress. These emotions, if not managed effectively, can further widen gaps in understanding and communication. As Dr. B highlighted, patients can "become very emotional and angry at the same time", especially if they believe they have missed an early diagnosis. When doctors discuss treatment options, patients may be overwhelmed by the influx of information.

The interviewees emphasized the need for empathy rather than a critical attitude towards patients and their families. Dr. C mentioned the need to provide reflective feedback through empathic dialogue and communication protocols, while Dr. B shared a practical approach by taking breaks. "We end the meeting and reassure the patient that it's okay to take some time, even a few days, to process what has happened. We fully understand and will arrange another meeting, perhaps the following week, when their carers and relatives will also be present. This will ensure that they have the support of the community and that there are others who can help them understand the situation."

Dr. E further pointed out the need to be prepared when making empathic responses. He suggested recognizing patients' emotions such as sadness, silence and shock, and understanding the causes and sources of these emotions. He stressed the importance of giving patients time to express their feelings and responding in a way that acknowledges their emotional state. Dr. D explained that doctors should recognise that during the onset of illness in critically ill patients, emotions can be very emotional and it is important to allow space for them to express themselves. It's noted that "we need to try to put ourselves in other people's shoes."

Barrier 3: Linguistic and Non-Verbal Communication Challenges

Communicating bad news involves both verbal and non-verbal elements, both crucial for conveying sensitive information. Dr. B pointed out that medical jargon often hinders effective communication, emphasizing the need to distill complex terminology into language patients can understand. This becomes particularly relevant when interacting with diverse patient demographics with varying levels of health literacy. Dr. A promoted tailored communication strategies that consider each patient's unique cognitive and sensory capabilities. She believes that such strategies can ensure that all patients, regardless of their background or condition, are equipped to make informed decisions about their illness.

Beyond verbal communication, the interviews also highlighted the importance of interpreting non-verbal cues. This is especially pertinent when interacting with patients who may have impairments affecting verbal expression, such as those resulting from a stroke or dementia. In these cases, effective communication depends heavily on clinician's ability to perceive and comprehend non-verbal signals, which makes the interaction a complex exercise in observation and interpretation (Dr. E).

Barrier 4: Effective Listening in Clinical Environment

The fourth barrier identied was the practical difficulty in engaging in active listening within the constraints of a high-pressure clinical environment. Participants stressed that listening is more than just hearing. It is a process requiring full presence, empathy, and understanding, yet it is often overlooked due to time pressures and administrative burdens on doctors (Dr. B, Dr. E). True listening, as one participant noted, is an active process of interpreting the underlying emotions and concerns behind a patient's or family's words, and the very start of good doctor-patient communication (Dr. E).

Participants advocated for a conscious shift in approach, urging doctors to set aside preconceived agendas and theoretical frameworks to truly understand the patient's experience (Dr. B). They suggested that the skill of active listening must be cultivated through practice in everyday personal interactions before it can be effectively deployed in high-stakes professional contexts. The inability to listen effectively was portrayed as fundamental impediment to all other communication efforts, which often leaves patients and families feeling unheard and compounding their distress.

Factors Underlying the Barriers

Paternalistic Mode of Communication

The paternalistic mode of communication, deeply rooted in collectivist cultures, presents a significant barrier to effective bad news delivery (Roman et al., 2013). In collectivist cultures like China, doctors are often seen as authoritative figures who prioritize decision-making over patient engagement, which can limit open communication (Liang et al., 2022). This hierarchical doctor-patient dynamic can discourage patients from expressing their concerns or asking questions, making it difficult for doctors to gauge their emotional state and provide the necessary empathy and support. This paternalistic approach assumes that doctors, due to their expertise, know what is best for the patient, which can lead to a lack of patient involvement in the decision-making process. Consequently, patients may feel disempowered and less likely to voice their concerns or preferences, which is crucial for accurate diagnosis and effective treatment.

In Chinese culture, the self-concept is deeply embedded within the family structure, contrasting markedly with the predominant individualistic ideas of Western cultures. The Chinese notion of self is intertwined with collective identity and the responsibilities that arise from familial roles. The emphasis on strong familial ties manifests in various forms but is particularly prominent in concepts like filial piety ('xiao'), which underscores the reverence and duty of children towards their parents (Zheng & Li, 2022). This concept is essential to understanding the psychological and emotional factors that emerge when confronting unfavorable health news. Filial piety dictates that adult children bear the responsibility of caring for their aging parents, a sentiment encapsulated in proverbs like "When a young bird grows up, it feeds its mother." Such sayings reflect a cultural expectation of reciprocal care, reinforcing the social obligation children feel towards their parents. In this context, the elderly are often viewed as fragile individuals, echoing the sentiment found in another proverb "treating the elders as if they were little kids." The perceived fragility of elderly parents compounds the emotional burden on their children when faced with serious health issues, compelling them to shield their parents from distressting information (Chi et al., 2018). This protective instinct can sometimes lead to misinformation or withholding of the truth, particularly in cases of illnesses like cancer, where bad news can be particularly burdensome for both the patient and their family. Adding to this complexity is the impact of China's one-child policy, which has had far-reaching social implications. The one-child policy, implemented in 1979 and relaxed officially in 2015, has led to a demographic landscape where many couples have only one child. As a result, the burden of caregiving and, by extension, the responsibility of conveying difficult information falls disproportionately on these single offspring. This singular responsibility can exacerbate feelings of stress and guilt if the treatment does not result in positive outcomes or if a parent's condition deteriorates.

Overwhelming Workloads in Hospitals

The high-pressure environment of a busy clinical setting in China can significantly impact the quality of delivering bad news to patients. Data showed that in 2015, physician density in urban China was about 3.8 per 1,000 people, while the density in rural areas remained consistently below 2 per 1,000 (Hsieh & Tang, 2019). Physicians in China often face overwhelming workloads and time constraints, leading to rushed conversations and missed opportunities for active listening. Wen et al. (2016) found that physicians typically work an average of 54.1 hours per week, with this heavy workload linked to various outcomes including declines in patient satisfaction and increased risk of burnout. Such long hours correlate with rushed interactions during patient consultations, where healthcare professionals have limited time to convey sensitive information adequately. This can make it challenging for doctors to provide the necessary empathy and support when delivering bad news in the oncology setting, such as a terminal diagnosis or the recurrence of a serious illness. In a typical Chinese hospital, three or more patients may share a single room, making private and in-depth conversations difficult. This lack of privacy can hinder the doctor's ability to communicate sensitive information effectively, leaving patients feeling unheard and misunderstood.

Lack of Corresponding Training

In China, many physicians and nurses in oncology settings lack the necessary skills for such communication, resulting in profound psychological impacts on patients and their families. A study conducted in a Beijing hospital targeting the clinical oncology setting (Pang et al., 2015) revealed that Chinese physicians find breaking bad news to be a highly stressful experience. Another study highlighted that while doctors may observe or receive instructions from senior colleagues on patient communication, they often lack structured training in essential communication skills, including breaking bad news (Hahne et al., 2020). The high-pressure environment in which healthcare providers operate often means that communication training is not prioritized. The approach for delivering bad news in China remains elusive and the existing methods are somehow untransferrable. Healthcare providers must navigate a delicate balance between disclosing cancer-related information and considering the patient's and family's needs. While Western practices emphasize patient autonomy, these concepts do not seamlessly translate to Asian cultures. In Chinese contexts, family decision-making holds paramount importance and is deeply intertwined with an individual's self-concept. The unique cultural context in which Chinese physicians operate necessitates that communication strategies be adapted. Culturally sensitive protocols can reportedly improve both the delivery of bad news and the overall patient experience (Wuensch et al., 2013).

Protocols of Breaking Bad News

Various strategies have been proposed to assist clinicians in delivering bad news. The SPIKES protocol, outlined by Baile et al. (2000), offers a structured approach for preparing doctors to communicate difficult information effectively. Numerous oncology practitioners find this standardized approach useful when initiating sensitive conversations. In the following, the mnemonic tool of SPIKES will be introduced. It is crucial to recognize that while protocols like SPIKES offers valuable guidance, cultural context plays a significant role. Healthcare providers should adapt their approach based on patients' cultural backgrounds rather than rigidly adhering to predefined steps. Also, individual preferences and expectations regarding bad news discussions can be influenced by factors such as gender, age, and the specific type of illness.

The Framework of SPIKES

S-Setting

The first step involves preparing mentally for the delivery of bad news, anticipating potential emotional reactions and difficult questions. It is important to create a private and focused environment, ensuring tissues are available, involving significant others at the patient's discretion, sitting down without barriers, establishing rapport through eye contact or touch, and managing time constraints and interruptions (Baile et al., 2000).

P-Perception

Before disclosing medical findings, clinicians should use open-ended questions to understand the patient's perception of their medical situation. This step helps correct any misinformation and tailor the conversation to the patient's level of understanding. It also identifies if the patient is in denial or has unrealistic expectations about their illness or treatment.

I-Invitation or Information

This step acknowledges that while most patients want full information about their condition, some may prefer not to know all the details. Clinicians should respect this coping mechanism and ask patients how they wish to receive information about test results or their condition. If a patient declines detailed information, clinicians can offer to answer future questions or discuss findings with a designated family member or friend.

K-Knowledge

Clinicians should gently warn patients before delivering bad news to help them brace for the impact. Communication should be clear, using layman's terms, avoiding technical jargon, and not overly blunt to prevent patient distress. Information should be given in manageable portions with regular checks for understanding. When prognosis is poor, it's important to convey that care continues with goals like pain control and symptom relief, rather than saying "nothing more can be done."

E-Empathy

Responding empathetically to a patient's emotions is crucial yet challenging. Clinicians should observe the patient's emotional cues, identify the emotion and its cause, and then connect with the patient by acknowledging their feelings. If emotions are not clearly expressed, exploratory questions can help clarify them. Empathic responses reduce feelings of isolation, offer support, and validate the patient's emotions as normal responses to their situation.

S-Summarize or Strategize

Creating a clear plan for the future can alleviate patient anxiety. Clinicians should ensure the patient is ready to discuss treatment plans, present options, and share decision-making responsibilities, which can help maintain the patient's sense of control and reduce physician feelings of failure when treatments are not successful. Addressing prognosis and treatment options, especially when unfavourable, requires sensitivity. Physicians should explore the patient's understanding, expectations, and fears to tailor discussions accordingly. Acknowledging patients' broader concerns and focusing on achievable goals like symptom management can provide reassurance and maintain hope.

The Application of SPIKES in the Chinese Context

In China, the adoption of communication protocols like SPIKES has become increasingly crucial. Research indicates a significant improvement in clinicians' ability to convey unfavorable diagnoses after implementing these protocols (Pang et al., 2015). Physicians report feeling more comfortable discussing diagnoses and end-of-life issues with patients and their families, without a corresponding increase in emotional distress (Wuensch et al., 2013). However, several challenges persist. First, it is essential to enhance communication by equipping medical students with discourse strategies that balance interpersonal skills and convey medical expertise (Pun, 2021). Since some students exhibit poor sensitivity to non-verbal cues, culturally appropriate training models for critical conversations should be promoted. Second, while the protocols are often directly adapted from the SPIKES model, tailoring these communication strategies to address the specific cultural and emotional needs of Chinese patients and their families remains essential. Cultural nuances, family dynamics, and patient expectations play a significant role in effective communication during difficult conversations (Hahne et al., 2020). Future investigations should delve deeper into adapting these protocols to the Chinese context. Third, the delivery of protocol education primarily occurs in major cities like Beijing and Hong Kong while the broader application of these strategies in regions with scarcer medical resources warrants further examination. Rural areas and smaller healthcare facilities face unique challenges, and ensuring consistent training and implementation across diverse settings is critical. Moreover, the workshops typically involve small-scale participation (often fewer than 100 attendees). While these workshops provide valuable insights, a more comprehensive understanding of their impact across a broader spectrum of healthcare providers and patients is yet to be fully explored.

Conclusion

In conclusion, this chapter underscores the significant impact of cultural and linguistic nuances when delivering difficult news, especially in the context of oncology. While the SPIKES protocol provides a valuable framework, its effectiveness hinges on thoughtful adaptation to China's distinct cultural context. Healthcare professionals face inherent challenges, but this chapter equips them with the necessary tools and knowledge to navigate these complexities with sensitivity and respect. Cultivating cultural competence is not just beneficial—it is essential for building trust and empathy in therapeutic relationships. As providers strive to communicate bad news compassionately and clearly, they must also honor the cultural values and emotional needs of Chinese cancer patients and their families. Integrating ethical communication with cultural insight reflects the holistic approach required in modern healthcare, addressing patients' medical, emotional, and cultural well-being.

Discussion Prompts

1. How do cultural values such as filial piety and collectivism influence the way bad news is communicated in Chinese oncology settings?
2. What are the major barriers to breaking bad news identified in this chapter, and how do they compare to those in Western contexts?
3. How can the SPIKES protocol be adapted to better suit the Chinese healthcare environment? What elements might need modification?
4. How do verbal and non-verbal communication interact in the delivery of bad news, and what role does language sensitivity play in this interaction?
5. To what extent does the paternalistic mode of communication still dominate doctor-patient interaction in Chinese medical institutions, and what are the implications for patient autonomy?

Reflection Questions

1. Reflect on a time when you or someone you know received difficult health news. How might cultural factors have shaped that experience?
2. What skills or training would you personally find most important in preparing for a conversation involving bad news in a multicultural setting?

3. What ethical tensions arise when a family requests that a cancer diagnosis not be disclosed to the patient? How would you respond in that situation?
4. How can empathy be demonstrated effectively in brief, high-pressure clinical encounters like those described in this chapter?
5. After reading this chapter, how might your communication style change when working with patients from cultures different from your own?

References

Baile, W. F., Buckman, R., Lenzi, R., Glober, G., Beale, E. A., & Kudelka, A. P. (2000). SPIKES-A six-step protocol for delivering bad news: Application to the patient with cancer. *The Oncologist, 5*(4), 302–311.

Buckman, R. (1992). *How to break bad news: A guide for health care professionals.* University of Toronto Press. 15.

Buckman, R. (1984). Breaking bad news: Why is it still so difficult. *British Medical Journal (Clinical Research Edition), 288*, 1597–1599.

Buckman, R. (1996). Talking to patients about cancer. *BMJ, 313*, 699–700.

Chi, H., Cataldo, J., Ho, E., & Rehm, R. (2018). Can we talk about it now? Recognizing the optimal time to initiate end-of-life care discussions with older chinese americans and their families. *Journal of Transcultural Nursing, 29*(6), 532–539.

Hsieh, C. R., & Tang, C. (2019). The multi-tiered medical education system and its influence on the health care market-China's Flexner Report. *Human Resources for Health, 17*(1), 50.

Kaplan, M. (2010). SPIKES: A framework for breaking bad news to patients with cancer. *Clinical Journal of Oncology Nursing, 14*(4), 514–516.

Liang, Z., Xu, M., Liu, G., Zhou, Y., & Howard, P. (2022). Patient-centred care and patient autonomy: Doctors' views in Chinese hospitals. *BMC Medical Ethics, 23*(1), 38.

Liu, Y., Yang, J., Huo, D., Fan, H., & Gao, Y. (2018). Disclosure of cancer diagnosis in China: The incidence, patients' situation, and different preferences between patients and their family members and related influence factors. *Cancer Management and Research*, 2173–2181.

Novack, D. H., Plumer, R., Smith, R. L., Ochitill, H., Morrow, G. R., & Bennett, J. M. (1979). Changes in physicians' attitudes toward telling the cancer patient. *JAMA, 241*(9), 897–900.

Pang, Y., Tang, L., Zhang, Y., Song, L., Goelz, T., Fritzsche, K., & Wuensch, A. (2015). Breaking bad news in China: Implementation and comparison of two communication skills training courses in oncology. *Psycho-Oncology, 24*(5), 608–611.

Parker, P. A., Baile, W. F., de Moor, C., Lenzi, R., Kudelka, A. P., & Cohen, L. (2001). Breaking bad news about cancer: Patients' preferences for communication. *Journal of Clinical Oncology, 19*(7), 2049–2056.

Pun, J. (2021). A study of Chinese medical students' communication pattern in delivering bad news: An ethnographic discourse analysis approach. *BMC Medical Education, 21*(1), 286.

Roman, G., Enache, A., Pârvu, A., Gramma, R., Moisa, ŞM., Dumitraş, S., & Ioan, B. (2013). Ethical issues in communication of diagnosis and end-of-life decision-making process in some of the Romanian Roma communities. *Medicine, Health Care, and Philosophy, 16*(3), 483–497.

Sweeny, K., Shepperd, J. A., & Han, P. K. J. (2011). The goals of communicating bad news in health care: Do physicians and patients agree? *Health Expectations, 14*(3), 230–238.

Tse, C. Y., Chong, A., & Fok, S. Y. (2003). Breaking bad news: A Chinese perspective. *Palliative Medicine, 17*(4), 339–343.

Wen, J., Cheng, Y., Hu, X., Yuan, P., Hao, T., & Shi, Y. (2016). Workload, burnout, and medical mistakes among physicians in China: A cross-sectional study. *Bioscience Trends, 10*(1), 27–33.

Wuensch, A., Tang, L., Goelz, T., Zhang, Y., Stubenrauch, S., Song, L., Hong, Y., Zhang, H., Wirsching, M., & Fritzsche, K. (2013). Breaking bad news in China—The dilemma of patients' autonomy and traditional norms. A first communication skills training for Chinese oncologists and caretakers. *Psychooncology, 5*(25), 1192–1195.

Zheng, X., & Li, H. (2022). How Chinese children's filial piety beliefs affect their parents' life satisfaction and loneliness. *Psych Journal, 11*(6), 863–872.

Chapter 5
A Narrative Approach to Comfort: Love Within Boundaries

Weiwei Lu

Introduction

This chapter explores the complexity of comforting cancer patients in emotionally charged situations, drawing on narrative practice to reflect on the ethical and emotional boundaries in clinician-patient communication. Through a case study encountered during fieldwork, it illustrates how oncologists, and those working closely with them, navigate the tension between professional detachment and emotional vulnerability in high-stakes medical encounters.

In Search of Comfort

On another ordinary day during my fieldwork for my PhD study, when I entered the medical oncology ward, a physician came to the department director, reporting a tough case.

A patient's son told the physician that he wanted to discharge his father from the hospital because they had a fight, and he wanted to give up his father's treatment. The physician told the department director that the patient was very emotional now and requested to talk with the Director. The Director went to the patient's room, trying to comfort him. I followed the Director and witnessed their conversation.

The original version of the chapter has been revised. A correction to this chapter can be found at https://doi.org/10.1007/978-981-96-9474-7_11

W. Lu (✉)
Department of Social and Behavioural Sciences, City University of Hong Kong, Hong Kong, China
e-mail: weiweilu6-c@my.cityu.edu.hk

J. Pun (ed.), *Teaching and Learning Oncology Communication*,
https://doi.org/10.1007/978-981-96-9474-7_5

The patient looked young, not yet over 60. He sat on the bed, complaining to the Director how his son disappointed him. He told the Director he wanted to talk to his son about his life stories, but the son did not want to listen. Then, he implicitly told his son that he would choose to commit suicide after he came back home from the hospital. His son did not empathize with him but responded to him that he dared not do that. His son's words irritated him, making him sad and angry.

The Director comforted him by saying that the son was still young, and he did not mean it, "You are a family, and he is your son. He will not be so cruel." However, the patient did not accept this reasoning and kept shaking his head. After the patient and the Director repeated several rounds of conversations, both became speechless. The Director spent half an hour talking to the patient. I stood beside the Director, witnessing his efforts to calm the patient and resolve his anger at his son. The patient desired the Director's listening; however, his emotion was not eased by the Director's words. Both tell the facts of the same event; both cannot understand each other. The Director is an experienced physician with over 20 years of clinical life. As an oncologist, his clinical motto is "seldom cure, often comfort." However, he admitted, it is much easier said than done.

How do we comfort cancer patients? This is a clinical challenge for all the healthcare professionals.

First, it is difficult for physicians to give "false hope" to patients (Eijkholt, 2020; Musschenga, 2019). The curability of cancer is a debate among physicians, which makes professionals hesitant to say to patients, "Everything will be fine." Second, physicians are trained to be rational on the facts of illness but lack the training to reconcile the objective disease with the subjective hope (Hancock et al., 2007). Third, physicians do not know how to comfort patients with emotional vulnerabilities (Ryan et al., 2005). When patients want to express their frustration, how to comfort them? When patients have depression, how to comfort them? When patients tend to commit suicide, how to comfort them? Moreover, family members also need comfort. How do physicians take care of family members?

Last, the difficulties in comforting patients will gradually erode physicians' energy. Physicians are human beings. When facing cancer patients' distress and pains, their instincts urge them to empathize and help patients. However, due to the helplessness accumulated through the failures of comforting patients, physicians face a higher chance of burnout. An alternative solution is to become numb to patients' hardships.

Thus, learning how to comfort patients is crucial for the high quality of healthcare and both physicians' and patients' well-being.

A Narrative Approach

The Director and the physician encouraged me to have a conversation with the patient. They introduced me to the patient as a psychologist, which implied that I was there to "comfort" him. I had to clarify my role as a researcher to the Director. Then, I invited the patient for an interview.

This case is much more complex beyond the emotional struggles in comforting patients. The patient is at the last stage of his life, making him very sensitive to others' reactions. Moreover, the Director told me the patient has intense conflicts with his family. He was very easy to be irritated and treated his wife violently. That's why only his son took care of him at the hospital. He also had a drug use history. He was not an obedient patient. Physicians warned him many times that he should quit smoking and was not allowed to take cigarettes in the ward, but he did not follow the rules. Apparently, this was a patient making the physician headache.

The complexity of this case was out of my expectations. This is not only because of the patient's rich and relatively "negative" experiences but also because of the implicit but desperate expectations from the patient and the physicians, hoping for me to solve this tough problem by providing a "counseling" session.

How Should I Prepare for This Interview?

The first thing is about positioning. I need to position myself in this conversation. As a narrative practitioner, I have conducted different kinds of narrative practice with old people in nursing homes, collective narratives with mothers, and online writing with all types of adult participants. As a narrative therapist, I help people find alternative understanding of their problems. As a narrative researcher, I am curious about how stories and storytelling influence people's knowledge and behaviors.

Though the patient and other physicians expect me to "solve" the problem, this is beyond my research ethics. However, in narrative practice, we learned that we should have conversations with persons as anthropologists with curiosity and openness (White, 1990). In this sense, the principle of narrative conversation is the same as qualitative research. As a researcher, I am responsible for listening to the patient without judgment and creating a safe space for him to share his stories and opinions. Therefore, I position myself as a researcher in our conversation. Second, I needed to collect more information about the patient. I had the diagnostic information and his emotional status from the Director. What else should I know? I did not know how many interviews we could have in the future. Then, I assumed we only had one conversation, which meant I needed to collect as much information as possible to prepare for the conversation. I heard there were conflicts between the patient and his family. So, I invited his son for a conversation to understand more about the situation. Surprisingly, the son shared with me that there was severe domestic violence in his family.

Third, I need to be aware of my bias and judgment. I was pretty shocked by the patient's behavior described by the son. Though the father admitted his history of drug use, he did not mention the part of domestic violence. I realized the "problem" was much more complicated than what had been told. I felt pity for the wife and the son. I could feel the son had tried his best to care for his father by upholding the responsibilities over his anger as a son. This interview was an ethical practice for me. On the one hand, I empathized with the son and the mother for the hardship they had experienced. On the other hand, I knew I needed to be aware of my biased empathy.

In narrative therapy, a fundamental claim is that the "problem is the problem. The person is not the problem." This statement requires us to understand the system that nurtures the problem, not to equal the person as the problem (White, 1990). When listening to the son, I tried to keep curious about the supporting system of the problem rather than seeing anyone in this system as a problem. The conversation with the son was like a warm-up narrative interview before the one with his father, which helped me keep my distance from emotions. I knew the only thing I should try my best to stick to was to listen to the patient attentively with curiosity.

Narrative Conversation

On the second day, I had a conversation with the patient.

When I entered the ward, the patient was sitting there, having an intravenous drip. He smiled at me, saying hi. I sat down beside his bed and began the interview by thanking him for having a chat with me about his cancer treatment decision-making experience. Then he started to tell his story.

Fifteen days ago, he went to the hospital for a cold. Then, he was diagnosed with cancer. His daughter brought him to this hospital, and he got the proper treatment in time. He was satisfied with the hospital and physicians. He said his problem was the conflict with family members, which made him feel bad. He was silent for a second when he said that.

I asked him, "Would you like to talk more about it?" This question unfolded the patient's sad story of a father.

The patient had six children, but he just kept the oldest daughter and the youngest son. Other children were given to his friends and relatives. Due to the one-child policy in China, he paid a lot of fines for extra children. He was a farmer at that time. Every year, he had to submit all the food he had planted for the punishment for each extra child. But that was not enough. He needed to sell all the valuable things to pay the money. Finally, he got a son. However, the punishment was continuous every year and made them unable to survive. Two times a year, when it was the harvest season, they would be asked to pay the fine. He had to take the whole family away from his hometown to make a living.

He went to many cities in China, running grocery shops, trading goods, and even being a security guard for parking lots. In the most difficult times, he worked three jobs daily.

When he mentioned he had six children, he started to sob. I was surprised by his emotional expression. But I immediately realized that he felt safe with me to share his deep sorrow. I felt sorry for his poor life experience. But at the same time, I know if I show my sympathy, if I say some words to comfort him, I would be in a judge's position to claim he had a worse life than others. While the patient's life story invited strong emotional responses, narrative practitioners are trained to withhold judgmental sympathy to avoid undermining the patient's agency and voice in constructing meaning. Otherwise, he may be placed in an inferior position and lose the confidence to share his story. I may interrupt his emotions and storyline. The conversation may end. Only when I keep curiosity and appreciate his resilience would I be able to explore the intrinsic motivation for his pursuit of a son.

So, I asked him, "Why so insisted on having a son?" He said, "In the countryside, if you do not have a son, you will be looked down upon by the family clan."

This belief motivated him to live around like a nomadic family for more than ten years. When he was 42, he decided to settle in the capital city of his home province. However, he said he was regretful for bringing his son to the city. The son was 8 years old when they started living in the city. He changed many schools because of behavioral issues. The father spent a lot of money each time to help him transfer schools. The most impressive memory was that his son was caught destroying the whole game center with the other three kids. The father gave him a sound beating. That incident made him reflect on his education for the son. He realized that his son did not know how to cherish the life he had. The son would fight with his parents if he could not get what he wanted. The son took expensive cigarettes that are eight times more than his father. He had to admit that he spoiled the son. It was a mistake that he brought his son to the city.

During our conversations, the father sighed almost every two sentences. I felt the same desperation as a parent when I listened to him. However, trained as a narrative practitioner, I should navigate emotions but not indulge in them and lose direction. I reminded myself I was interviewing with this patient. It was neither an ordinary chat nor a counseling session. I would like to know more about this patient's treatment decision-making trajectory. In storytelling, strong emotions easily attract or overwhelm us (Jasper, 1998; Maslach, 2018; Norman, 2002). However, emotions are entrances to the core values of this person. Why do people have emotions? Because something triggers the things that matter to them.

To open the story behind the emotion, I asked the patient, "Did you accept your son being grown up in this way?" The patient said yes.

He then talked about more accidents of his son, costing a lot of money and energy to cope with. He even mentioned his dissatisfaction with his wife's education to the son, which was very ineffective. He summarized that it was retribution to him.

If I had not had a conversation with the patient's son first, I would have been persuaded by the patient's story and felt unfair for this father. This is a pitfall of narrative, which is often challenged by its authenticity (Shapiro, 2011). In narrative practice training, we do not judge the authenticity of a narrative. We choose to trust the authenticity of the story. One reason is that there will be no collaboration in solving the problem if there is no trust. Another reason is the narrative is co-constructed by the interlocutors as co-authors. We should believe in the stories that are co-constructed by ourselves. As an interviewer, I was also responsible for this story. My contribution to this story is represented in my positioning in this conversation, my questions to the teller, and my responses to the sharer's various kinds and levels of expressions (Cremin et al., 2018; Taylor et al., 2007).

Therefore, I tried to encourage the patient to reflect on his life rather than engage in negative moods. I asked him, "Why do you call it retribution?" The patient was surprised by my question and answered, "Don't you think so too?" "I mean, it sounds like you did something bad first, then received the consequence."

It was bold for me to challenge a vulnerable patient. Many people, like physicians, family members, and any other people, ill people are regarded as weak. However, in narrative practice, we respect that every person has hopes and dreams, skills, and abilities to deal with the problems that have trapped them deeply (White, 1990, 2007).

People are sick, but it does not mean they are weak. In contrast, during my interviews with other cancer patients, I heard many "hero" stories about how they survived the hardships in life and how they survived painful cancer treatment. The empowerment of patients is not only to amplify their voices but also to polish their strengths and identities to eliminate the social prejudice of "the sick role" (Aujoulat et al., 2008).

The patient murmured about previously punishing his son harshly, hinting at deeper familial tensions. This moment revealed a narrative gap—common in clinical encounters—where a patient's version of events omits painful or shameful truths, underscoring the challenges of emotional engagement in narrative interviews.

In narrative practice, we should be aware that every narrative has gaps (Frank, 2010). These gaps are the pathways to alternative stories, or multiple stories intersected in the same event (Bolaki, 2016; White, 1990).

When the patient mentioned the "retribution," I was curious whether it would be a bridge to enter the patient's alternative narrative of the family relationship. However, he "refused" to move forward in this way.

He was irritated and said he would like to stop the conversation. I felt a moment of embarrassment and made efforts to distract him by asking other questions.

He continued answering my questions, disclosing his wish to have normal conversations with his son and family as ordinary families do. He could not understand why his input in the family did not win the respect and gratitude of the son but only complaints. He wished his son to accept him as he had accepted the son.

I could not help him. It was not ethical for me to say that the reason might be his violence towards his wife and son that made the divide between them. That was my judgment, not the patient's knowledge concluded through his telling. In our conversation, we did not touch on anything about domestic violence. When we were at the edge of that violent aspect, the patient lost patience. He was not ready for exploration. Instead, he told me, "You did not understand what bothers me. You are not a qualified doctorate."

I politely responded to him that I needed to learn more. Then, we ended the conversation for him to take more rest.

Narrative "Therapy"

I knew I did not aim to comfort this cancer patient because I positioned myself as a researcher to have an interview with him. However, I felt slightly frustrated that I did not meet his expectations during our conversation. And I had to admit that I got a little bit hurt by his denial words that shook my confidence and identity as a novice researcher.

I believe a lot of junior physicians experienced the same frustration as me.

When we have narrative conversations, we need to create a safe space for each other because we are vulnerable in sincere sharing. It is just like a tango; we must collaborate to avoid stepping on another's feet. However, the reality is we often "get our feet stepped on" in the communication between physicians and patients.

Experiencing the conversation with this patient, I understood why physicians feared talking to him. It is easy to get "hurt." And now it was my turn. Many physicians choose to let go without deconstructing the problem and strengthening their confidence from them. Physicians are busy doing different kinds of tasks every day. Ignoring these subtle feelings seems the most effective way to deal with this issue. However, we all know that as time goes by, these little things will lead to the deterioration of physicians' mental health.

How can I get rid of this disempowerment, though it was not so significant?

The most important thing for me was whether I performed my ethical responsibility as a researcher. At the very beginning, I positioned this conversation as a research interview, and I applied the proper attitude as an interviewer. When the patient shared his tears and thoughts with me, he was safe and comfortable to do that. Throughout the conversation, I listened to him attentively, following his words to inquire about more details. I was aware of the patient's emotions and behaviors. When he was not ready for the exploration, I followed his choice. Most importantly, I did not intervene to solve his problems.

In this way, the patient felt disappointed because he expected me to comfort him. But what I did was just listening to him with full respect. Though the patient claimed I was not so professional, I think I was professional because I was not involved in his improper expectations.

This experience made me realize that physicians might experience these struggles many times each day. When patients are desperate, lonely, or depressed, they are inclined to depend on healthcare professionals to solve their problems, including physical and mental distress (Cain et al., 2018). However, not all physicians can command the boundary of comfort. Physicians may become emotional labors (Larson & Yao, 2005), developing their abilities to provide humanistic care by unconsciously taking the risk of burnout or becoming medical experts who are good at fixing "medical problems." However, most physicians struggle in between.

Mutual Empowerment

With the progress of my fieldwork, I gradually forgot the spiciness of the conversation between me and the patient. Two weeks later, when I was walking in the hospital, I saw a wheelchair rolling toward me, and the patient sitting in it was just him! He was also surprised to see me too. But immediately, we both smiled and greeted each other! I never forgot his expression. His eyes brightened with a relaxing smile when he recognized me, like meeting an old friend!

I promised him I would visit him in the ward again. Then, we had a second conversation.

I thought I had got rid of his straightforward comments about me, but I felt so relieved when he smiled at me when we met accidentally.

When I entered his room, he sat on the bed waiting for me. When he saw me, he gently bowed his upper body and said "Thank you" to me! That behavior made me truly touched. I also noticed another surprise. His wife was taking care of him. He was calm and obedient with her around.

It was much more relaxing to start the conversation than last time. I heard from the physicians that he came to the hospital because his condition got worse. But when we talked, he looked energetic and as articulate as usual. I never regarded him as a dying person. So did he.

This time, I did not prepare any questions. He had a lot to say. Many points he shared had become the motivation for my research work.

> "No matter rich or poor people, they struggle in this world. Once they lie on this bed, they will have the desire to live, which becomes the source of mental illness. Because they want to survive and see the bigger world, they will become more self-centered and depressed. You (counselors) need to carefully understand this psychological mechanism of patients."

> "If patients can open their hearts to express their feelings and sufferings, the power of healing is much stronger than the physical treatment. They may be unable to walk and sit, but they will be full of energy."

> "To better care for patients' mental health, we must educate physicians and nurses properly. They are the persons getting the closest access to patients. Patients will benefit most if the overall quality of humanistic care is improved. However, depending on a small number of clinical counselors in each department, it will not be helpful in general."

> "We need a systematic design of care for patients' physical and mental health. When a patient has a disease, how to talk to them is very important. If there is a conflict, how to deal with it? The same word and sentence will carry different meanings if they are spoken in different tones and methods."

> "About quitting smoking, I have my reason. I once successfully quit my drug addiction, which demonstrated that I had a strong will to change a habit. Why can I not quit smoking? Physicians should care about my reasoning, not just suggesting that I quit immediately and completely. In my village, there was a person who got the same disease as me. But he kept smoking and lived for 13 years after diagnosis. Physicians may suggest me to quit smoking gradually while listening to me about my resistance."

I never imagined I could learn so much from a drug taker, a violent husband, a poor farmer, a small business boss, a parking lot security guard, a bad-temper patient, and a dying person.

However, what made me feel sad was that no one in the hospital or his family ever listened to him.

This is not a unique case. During my fieldwork, a nurse also shared a story of her patient, whom all his family members hated, but the nurse saw the good side of this patient as a person.

It was a pity that many people died without resolving the poor relationships with their family members. Due to the disease's rapid progress or the problem's complexity, they failed to relieve the family entanglements. Thus, the disease left many unmet wishes and regrets for the patients and their families. However, healthcare professionals are the strangers who take care of their bodies, having the advantage of seeing their vulnerabilities and empowering them to be better by helping them construct their stories.

Comfort as Love within Boundaries

Soon after, I shared the interaction between me and this patient in a speech for over 200 of the physicians and nurses in the hospital. We all know cancer patients need comfort, but what does comfort mean?

From a narrative approach, comfort means the endeavors to create a safe space for the patients, unfolding their stories and witnessing the power of life in their stories.

Every person is suffering in this world. Thus, every person has the strength to survive their sufferings. We should respect their resilience in these sufferings, appreciate the dreams and hopes behind the resilience, and learn the skills and abilities from them to enrich our knowledge.

Everyone needs others to witness their willpower in distress and acknowledge their efforts in coping with difficulties. Through telling their stories, they reorganized the meaning of their lives and acquired evidence of their existence in this world. As people who listen and respond to these stories, we are the co-authors of their stories and identities (Albrecht et al., 2008; Eggly, 2002; Kalitzkus & Matthiessen, 2009).

Thus, for patients, the comfort is being heard, witnessed, appreciated, and acknowledged by others through the co-construction of their stories.

Narrative conversations can provide us with adequate communication skills to comfort patients. First, we should develop our curiosity. Everyone has a story. What is it? How does it influence patients' health and the relevant treatment decisions? When we value the importance of life stories in understanding patients, we will be motivated to listen to their stories. Second, we should see patients as equal to us. Though patients have diseases, they are human beings as strong as us, or even stronger and braver if we understand how painful the cancer treatment process they need to go through. Third, we should be non-judgmental. If I had a negative judgment of the patient after I knew his experience of domestic violence, drug addiction, and resistance to treatment, I would not be able to talk to him with curiosity. Thus, we must train ourselves to be aware of our values and the possible bias against patients, learn to put aside our biased judgment (including empathy), and keep an open attitude toward the uncertain interaction with patients.

Last, as the co-authors of patients' stories, we should fulfill our responsibilities to help them construct their stories. Patients come to hospitals with their "broken stories" because the disease disrupts their everyday life (Brody, 1994). When patients share their stories with us, they hope the listeners can "fix" their stories. We can listen to them attentively and ask follow-up questions to encourage them to elaborate more details. We can also catch every highlight in their life course or treatment process and celebrate each small achievement to develop a positive side of the story.

No matter how many skills we have, it is always hard to comfort patients. Because to comfort is to love. How do you love a strange, fragile, and even offensive person? The fundamental dilemma of institutionalized rationality in medical professionalism and the instinct of care in humanity makes love challenging for every healthcare professional (Rhodes, 2020).

However, we must learn to care for them. This is our responsibility and morality. What we should do is love patients within a certain boundary.

During my fieldwork, many physicians shared with me their issues of burnout. Being regarded as rational authorities, they should hold their personal feelings inside. All the frustration and anger brought by inefficient or ineffective communication with patients, caregivers, or other professionals will lead to burnout and moral distress (Sorensen & Iedema, 2009; Trufelli et al., 2008; Ulrich & Grady, 2023). For oncologists who also deal with patients' deaths, they need more emotional support from institutional and healthcare systems.

However, physicians have nowhere to digest their emotions. Physicians told me they did not share emotions with colleagues. They chose to drink or talk with friends outside the workplace to relieve the stress or sadness. They said if they shared the difficulties in communication with patients, they would be laughed at as poor physicians who couldn't control or manage patients. Thus, physicians do not discuss how to improve communication skills with each other.

This is not rare in this department and this hospital. Physicians' mental health is an international concern in healthcare systems (Cho & Huang, 2020; Hlubocky et al., 2016). We as physicians focus much more on improving our communication skills to comfort patients while too much less on how to comfort ourselves.

Thus, my interview case here may provide some references for physicians to apply in their communication with patients.

First, be clear about the boundary in each conversation. What roles and responsibilities you need to perform in the conversation as a physician? Is it a conversation about treatment options of surgery or chemotherapy? Is it a conversation about the treatment or emotion? When the content varies, the roles and responsibilities vary too. Physicians can position themselves to prepare for conversations.

Second, be open to the resistance in the conversations. Resistance makes us uncomfortable. However, resistance is a sign of engagement and a sense of safety, which means patients feel comfortable expressing their feelings and opinions. Moreover, resistances demonstrate the implicit preferences behind the disagreement or distraction. Physicians can follow with the resistance to explore what really matters to patients (Koenig, 2011).

Third, take care of yourself in time. The whole universe knows physicians are swamped every day. However, it should not be the reason for neglecting feelings and reactions to interactions and communication with patients. Physicians should gain the ability to deconstruct the frustration in their communication with patients and grow their resilience and wisdom from every small hurdle to avoid the accumulation of negative emotions.

Last, patients are also the co-authors of physicians' professional stories. Without patients' input, physicians' stories cannot move on. Thus, every conversation is an unknown journey in which physicians and patients co-construct a coherent story to support physicians and patients to be the persons they want to be. Physicians can change their perspectives to love patients as equal co-authors, relieving them from the uncomfortable power imbalance in the physician and patient role set.

Thus, by taking care of themselves through good preparation for the conversation, an effective management of boundaries in the conversation, and a timely reflection after the conversation, physicians can take good care of themselves and comfort patients within boundaries.

To conclude, this case exemplifies the emotional labour inherent in oncology communication and highlights the power of narrative approaches in fostering patient trust and dignity. By adopting a stance of non-judgmental listening and reflective positioning, healthcare professionals can offer comfort while protecting their own well-being—an essential theme echoed throughout this volume. Such narrative encounters challenge professionals to reframe their role not just as medical providers, but as co-authors in the patient's final chapters of life.

Discussion Prompts

1. How does the chapter define "comfort" in the context of physician–patient relationships, and how is this understanding shaped by narrative practice?
2. What ethical tensions arise when researchers or clinicians are expected to provide emotional support during interviews or consultations?
3. How can narrative approaches help health professionals maintain appropriate emotional boundaries while still demonstrating empathy?
4. What does this chapter reveal about the challenges of emotional labor and burnout among oncologists?
5. How might the narrative tools discussed here be integrated into communication training for healthcare professionals, particularly in end-of-life care?

Reflection Questions

1 Have you ever experienced or witnessed a situation where emotional expectations conflicted with professional boundaries? How was it handled?

2 Reflect on the idea that "the problem is the problem, the person is not the problem." How might this narrative principle shift your approach to challenging patients or families?
3 How do power dynamics between patients and clinicians influence the storytelling and meaning-making processes in medical encounters?
4 What strategies can clinicians adopt to protect their own mental health when dealing with emotionally charged conversations?
5 How might you personally apply the concept of "comfort as love within boundaries" in your own practice or professional context?

References

Albrecht, T. L., Eggly, S. S., Gleason, M. E. J., Harper, F. W. K., Foster, T. S., Peterson, A. M., Orom, H., Penner, L. A., & Ruckdeschel, J. C. (2008). Influence of clinical communication on patients' decision making on participation in clinical trials. *Journal of Clinical Oncology : Official Journal of the American Society of Clinical Oncology, 26*(16), 2666–2673. https://doi.org/10.1200/JCO.2007.14.8114

Aujoulat, I., Marcolongo, R., Bonadiman, L., & Deccache, A. (2008). Reconsidering patient empowerment in chronic illness: A critique of models of self-efficacy and bodily control. *Social Science & Medicine, 66*(5), 1228–1239.

Bolaki, S. (2016). *Illness as many narratives: Arts, medicine and culture*. Edinburgh University Press.

Brody, H. (1994). "My story is broken; can you help me fix it?": Medical ethics and the joint construction of narrative. *Literature and Medicine, 13*(1), 79–92.

Cain, C. L., Surbone, A., Elk, R., & Kagawa-Singer, M. (2018). Culture and palliative care: Preferences, communication, meaning, and mutual decision making. *Journal of Pain and Symptom Management, 55*(5), 1408–1419.

Cho, H. L., & Huang, C. J. (2020). Why mental health–related stigma matters for physician wellbeing, burnout, and patient care. *Journal of General Internal Medicine, 35*, 1579–1581.

Cremin, T., Flewitt, R., Swann, J., Faulkner, D., & Kucirkova, N. (2018). Storytelling and story-acting: Co-construction in action [Article]. *Journal of Early Childhood Research, 16*(1), 3–17. https://doi.org/10.1177/1476718X17750205

Eggly, S. (2002). Physician-patient co-construction of illness narratives in the medical interview [Article]. *Health Communication, 14*(3), 339–360. https://doi.org/10.1207/S15327027HC1403_3

Eijkholt, M. (2020). Medicine's collision with false hope: The false hope harms (FHH)argument. *Bioethics, 34*(7), 703–711.

Frank, A. W. (2010). *Letting stories breathe: A socio-narratology*. University of Chicago Press.

Hancock, K., Clayton, J. M., Parker, S. M., der Wal, S., Butow, P. N., Carrick, S., Currow, D., Ghersi, D., Glare, P., & Hagerty, R. (2007). Truth-telling in discussing prognosis in advanced life-limiting illnesses: A systematic review. *Palliative Medicine, 21*(6), 507–517.

Hlubocky, F. J., Back, A. L., & Shanafelt, T. D. (2016). Addressing burnout in oncology: Why cancer care clinicians are at risk, what individuals can do, and how organizations can respond. *American Society of Clinical Oncology Educational Book, 36*, 271–279.

Jasper, J. M. (1998). The emotions of protest: Affective and reactive emotions in and around social movements. *Sociological Forum, 13*(3).

Kalitzkus, V., & Matthiessen, P. F. (2009). Narrative-based medicine: Potential, pitfalls, and practice. *The Permanente Journal, 13*(1), 80.

Koenig, C. J. (2011). Patient resistance as agency in treatment decisions. *Social Science & Medicine, 72*(7), 1105–1114.
Larson, E. B., & Yao, X. (2005). Clinical empathy as emotional labor in the patient-physician relationship. *JAMA, 293*(9), 1100–1106.
Maslach, C. (2018). Burnout: A multidimensional perspective. In *Professional burnout* (pp. 19–32). CRC Press.
Musschenga, B. (2019). Is there a problem with false hope? *The Journal of Medicine and Philosophy: A Forum for Bioethics and Philosophy of Medicine, 44*(4).
Norman, D. (2002). Emotion & design: attractive things work better. *Interactions, 9*(4), 36–42.
Rhodes, R. (2020). *The trusted doctor: Medical ethics and professionalism.* Oxford University Press.
Ryan, H., Schofield, P., Cockburn, J., Butow, P., Tattersall, M., Turner, J., Girgis, A., Bandaranayake, D., & Bowman, D. (2005). How to recognize and manage psychological distress in cancer patients. *European Journal of Cancer Care, 14*(1), 7–15.
Shapiro, J. (2011). Illness narratives: Reliability, authenticity and the empathic witness. *Medical Humanities, 37*, 68–72.
Sorensen, R., & Iedema, R. (2009). Emotional labour: Clinicians' attitudes to death and dying. *Journal of Health Organization and Management, 23*(1), 5–22.
Taylor, K., Durant, R., & Boje, D. (2007). Telling the story, hearing the story: Narrative co-construction and crisis research [Article]. *American Communication Journal, 9*(1). https://www.scopus.com/inward/record.uri?eid=2-s2.0-38549179345&partnerID=40&md5=fd2004a67ff30690f8e3938e38805267
Trufelli, D., Bensi, C., Garcia, J., Narahara, J., Abrão, M., Diniz, R., Da Costa Miranda, V., Soares, H., & Del Giglio, A. (2008). Burnout in cancer professionals: A systematic review and meta-analysis. *European Journal of Cancer Care, 17*(6), 524–531.
Ulrich, C. M., & Grady, C. (2023). Measuring moral distress and its various sources. *The American Journal of Bioethics, 23*(4), 63–65.
White, M. (1990). *Narrative means to therapeutic ends* (1st ed.). Norton.
White, M. K. (2007). *Maps of narrative practice.* WW Norton & Company.

Chapter 6
Navigating Cultural Sensitivities: Communication in End-Of-Life Care for Chinese Cancer Patients

Kexin Tan

Chapter Summary
End-of-life (EOL) communication is a cornerstone of palliative care, particularly poignant in the context of Chinese cancer patients. These crucial conversations serve as a conduit for expressing treatment expectations, final wishes, and the myriad challenges faced during this vulnerable phase of life. Such open and honest dialogues are instrumental in facilitating a "good death," where patients are afforded dignity and peace in their final moments. The ripple effect of these interactions offers comfort and a sense of closure to caregivers, who are integral to the patient's support system. This chapter specifically addresses the complexities and cultural intricacies of EoL communication with Chinese cancer patients. In a society where traditional values deeply influence perceptions of illness and mortality, these discussions are laden with cultural significance. The convergence of ancient philosophies and contemporary medical ethics presents a unique set of challenges for healthcare providers. They must tread carefully, balancing the need for clear medical guidance with the cultural sensitivities that shape the patient's and family's experience. As we navigate through this chapter, we will explore how EoL communication can be tailored to respect the cultural context of Chinese cancer patients, ensuring that their journey towards life's end is met with understanding, compassion, and culturally congruent care. Through this focused lens, we aim to provide healthcare professionals with insights and strategies that honour both the medical and cultural needs of Chinese cancer patients at the end of life.

K. Tan (✉)
Department of English and Communication, The Hong Kong Polytechnic University, Hong Kong, China
e-mail: kexin.tan@connect.polyu.hk

J. Pun (ed.), *Teaching and Learning Oncology Communication*,
https://doi.org/10.1007/978-981-96-9474-7_6

Introduction

The end-of-life (EoL) phase is an essential yet often neglected aspect of healthcare. This period, typically the last 6–12 months of life, is associated with significant preventable suffering (Hui et al., 2014). Projections indicate that by 20642060, serious health-related suffering at EoL will nearly double from 26 million in 2016 to 48 million (Sleeman et al., 2019). Upper middle-income countries like China are expected to see an 87% increase in such suffering (Sleeman et al., 2019). Given these impending challenges and China's substantial contribution to global cancer statistics–24.1% of the world's new cancer cases and 26.5% of cancer deaths in 2022 (Bray et al., 2024; Han et al., 2024)–there has been an intensified focus on improving EoL care. The Chinese government's establishment of hospice care guidelines in 2017 marked an important step. The subsequent expansion of the program to an additional 71 areas by 2019 further demonstrates a strong commitment to addressing these needs (Yan et al., 2020).

Effective EoLC plays a pivotal role in the quality of cancer care provided during a patient's final days. EoLC informs patients and families about medical conditions and treatments, facilitating informed decision-making and preparation for the end-of-life phase (PDQ, 2024). Through these conversations, healthcare providers can better understand and respect the final wishes of patients, ensuring that care is personalized and aligns with preferred ways of being cared for (Maubach et al., 2019). This mutual understanding between patients and clinicians regarding treatment expectations and budget constraints can often result in more cost-effective medical care (Luta et al., 2021). Acknowledging patients' emotional responses, healthcare providers can offer a more holistic care experience that prevents patients from feeling abandoned. Furthermore, effective EoLC enables healthcare providers to administer appropriate medical interventions that not only improve the quality of life for patients nearing death but also extend consideration to the emotional well-being of caregivers. Active involvement in EoLC reduces caregivers' risk of depression post-bereavement (Wright et al., 2010).

In practice, however, EoLC does not always meet its intended goals. Studies reveal that critical discussions about future care preferences are frequently postponed until patients are in rapid decline, impeding effective dialgoue and agreement among family members (Pun, 2020). Healthcare professionals may neglect to communicate that a patient is approaching the end of life. This often leads to inadequate care planning and a lack of informed discussions about the patient's desires, contributing to overoptimism (Miller et al., 2022). Communication between staff, patients, and their families can be insufficient, resulting in misunderstandings and unclear expectations about prognosis and care options (Hagerty et al., 2005).

In Chinese culture, EoLC is influenced by Confucian values, which emphasize family-centered decision-making and often involve withholding prognostic information to protect the patient's emotional well-being (Jeon & Jing, 2023). This approach contrasts with Western expectations of individual autonomy and informed consent. The cultural nuances of EoLC in Chinese society merit further attention in academic research and practical application to ensure culturally sensitive care that respects both patient autonomy and family roles.

This chapter explores the complexities and cultural intricacies of EoL communication with Chinese cancer patients, investigating how Confucian ethics shape family dynamics and decision-making processes. It begins with a foundational understanding of EoLC through theoretical and operational definitions, setting the stage for an in-depth analysis of China's current EoLC landscape. The chapter then moves to the cultural norms underpinning EoLC, particularly Confucianism and relational autonomy, which significantly influence decision-making at the end of life. Through vivid scenarios and insightful interviews with family members and oncologists, the chapter illuminates the multifaceted experiences surrounding EoLC in China. It concludes with actionable suggestions for improving EoLC practices, such as conducting family meetings and enhancing healthcare providers' communication skills that honor both familial roles and patient autonomy.

Theoretical and Operation Definition of EoLC

End-of-life Care (EoLC) is defined by the Institute of Medicine (IoM) as "a process that addresses the comprehensive needs of patients nearing the end of life, including medical, social, emotional, and spiritual aspects" (2015). It typically includes a spectrum of services from disease-specific treatments to palliative and hospice care. EoLC primarily targets patients in the terminal phase, while palliative care can be provided at any stage of a serious illness, focusing on pain and symptom control alongside curative treatments. EoLC adopts a holistic approach that equally values the social, emotional, and spiritual well-being of patients.

The operational definition of EoLC, while comprehensive, prompts critical considerations about its practical application. Determining the appropriate scope of EoLC involves identifying which services are most beneficial at different stages of a terminal illness (Bhadelia et al., 2022). This includes not only medical interventions but also support for emotional and spiritual needs, which may evolve as the patient's condition progresses. The timing of EoLC implementation is equally crucial; it should be introduced at a point where it can provide maximum benefit and quality of life for the patient (Walczak, et al., 2017). This requires a dynamic and responsive approach from healthcare providers, who must continuously assess and adjust care plans in accordance with the patient's changing needs and wishes. Ultimately, the operational definition of EoLC must be flexible enough to accommodate individual circumstances while upholding its goal of providing holistic and compassionate care (Egan & Labyak, 2006).

EoLC in China

Before delving into the cultural dimensions of EoLC in China, it is essential to first examine the current situation that shapes its practices across mainland China, Hong Kong, and Macau. In China, the preference for the place of death is shaped by a multifaceted policy landscape. The distribution of opioid pain medication is stringently controlled outside hospitals, which is in stark contrast to policies in the United States, where home deaths are more common due to improved access to pain management. Additionally, hospital inpatient services receive higher reimbursement rates from China's social health insurance schemes, incentivizing patients to opt for continued treatment in hospitals rather than entering EoLC programs (Chen et al., 2023). Shanghai stands out as the only city where social insurance covers palliative care services, creating a more supportive environment for EoLC (Gong & Bai, 2022). In 2017 and 2019, significant strides were made with the launch of hospice care pilot programs across various regions, yet the responsibility for providing care remains mainly in the hands of doctors and hospitals (Cong, 2022).

In Hong Kong, public hospitals' acute medical and surgical wards are not conducive to a quality EoL experience. Specialty EoL services in Hong Kong public hospitals are limited and face referral challenges (Yee et al., 2020). Despite an increase in hospice beds, demand continues to exceed supply. Non-governmental organizations (NGOs), including Residential Care Homes for the Elderly (RCHEs), struggle with providing high-quality EoL care due to inadequately equipped facilities and a lack of personalized care (Chung & Yeoh, 2019). The private sector offers higher quality EoL services but at a cost that is less accessible to poorer populations (Luk et al., 2011).

Macao's palliative care development lags behind its aging population's needs and high life expectancy. The healthcare infrastructure is insufficient to support diverse healthcare needs. The first hospice, established in 2000, was initially limited to terminal cancer patients until its expansion in 2019. Despite a government action plan launched in 2016 aimed at improving community end-of-life care, there have been no specific goals or evaluations to measure its effectiveness, leading to a disconnect between policy intentions and actual service provision (The Macao SAR Government).

Reflecting on the current EoLC situation, which is characterized by stringent policies, limited access to pain management, and infrastructural challenges, we can see how these factors not only shape healthcare practices but also intersect with and influence cultural norms surrounding EoL decisions among Chinese patients. We now turn to explore how cultural norms specifically influence EoL decisions among Chinese cancer patients.

Cultural Norms

Cultural norms significantly influence EoL expectations in China, where it is customary for patients to defer critical EoL treatment decisions to their physicians. These medical professionals often consider the family's perspective, particularly that of adult children, when making decisions. Rooted in cultural norms, physicians typically consult with the patient's family before communicating severe or terminal diagnoses to the patient. For instance, a survey in Shandong province revealed that 98% of physicians would discuss cancer diagnoses with the family first, and 82% would refrain from informing the patient if the family wished so (Wang et al., 2018). Similarly, in Changsha, studies indicate that physicians tend to have separate conversations about palliative care with family members and patients, being more transparent with family members regarding prognosis and care objectives. These practices underscore an ethical dilemma for physicians who must balance respecting the family's wish to protect the patient from a distressing cancer diagnosis against upholding the patient's right to informed decision-making regarding their palliative care (Hahne et al., 2022).

This deference to family in medical decision-making is deeply intertwined with the Confucian value of filial piety, which profoundly impacts medical information disclosure in Chinese society. Filial piety mandates children's respect, obedience, and support towards their parents, encompassing honouring ancestors and preserving the family lineage. In healthcare, this value system leads families to often take on the role of decision-makers for medical care, asserting it as their natural right. As a result, families may opt to withhold medical information from patients as a means of protection and as part of their duty to ensure parents' longevity and well-being—a testament to the family's proper care (Jeon & Jing, 2023).

Building on this cultural foundation, recent findings by Leng et al. (2022) suggest a gradual shift towards a more patient-centered approach in EoLC. While extending life remains a priority for patients with terminal cancer, there is growing attention on improving quality of life during EoLC and supporting home deaths. These findings advocate for open communication about care preferences and informed choices as essential elements for enhancing EoL care outcomes. This emerging healthcare perspective does not conflict with but rather expands upon filial piety's principles by broadening its scope to include not only life preservation but also quality enrichment during life's final stages.

Amidst this changing landscape of EoLC, the notion of relational autonomy has become increasingly salient. This notion, which views patient autonomy as being shaped by familial and social ties, is gaining traction in modern bioethics. It questions the longstanding bioethical stance against medical paternalism and resonates with the philosophical insights of Paul Ricoeur (Ricoeur, 1992). According to Ricoeur, an individual's sense of self and autonomy emerge from the interactions with their social and cultural milieu. This philosophical viewpoint emphasizes that personal autonomy is not merely an isolated self-governance but is deeply interconnected with one's social environment and interpersonal bonds. When it comes to making decisions at the end of life, this philosophical idea implies that patients' choices are shaped by their engagement with family members, healthcare providers, and prevailing cultural values. It calls for a decision-making process that respects the patient's autonomy while also integrating the perspectives and support of their social network. This method acknowledges the importance of joint dialogue in EoLC, ensuring that decisions reflect both the patient's wishes and the collective wisdom of their trusted relationships.

In China, where the self is seen through a Confucian lens as inherently social, the concept of relational autonomy is especially relevant. Research by Cheng et al. (2021) supports this view, showing that a significant majority of cancer patients (65.7%) wish to be informed about their diagnosis or prognosis. Additionally, over half (54%) place a higher value on improving their quality of life rather than extending it, and a substantial portion are at ease with family members making medical decisions on their behalf. These findings highlight the profound impact of familial relationships on medical decision-making in China. The next section will delve into a specific EoLC scenario in China, examining how deeply rooted cultural values inform patient care and influence decision-making at life's end.

Scenario 1: At the Crossroads of Love and Loss-As Family Member of the Patient

(This scenario is a composite narrative based on a case provided by oncologiest Dr. Sunny Kong to illustrate the emotional and cultural complexities of end-of-life care.) *"I never imagined life without him," Mrs. X wept, gazing at her husband, Mr. X, who had been bedridden for months since his brain tumour haemorrhage. After the surgery to remove part of his skull, a tracheostomy, and a feeding tube, he lay there with open eyes, but it was unclear how much of him remained. The tumour had not only consumed his brain but also the future of this young couple, married for only a few years.*

Ourpalliative care team was called in as Mr. X suffered more frequent infections and seizures. The chances of starting any oncological treatment safely were grim. Amidst the beeping of medical monitors, Mrs. X continued, "No one will ever love,value, or understand me as much as he does".

Every day, Mrs. X was at the ward entrance, waiting for visiting hours. She spent every moment, aside from sleep, by her husband's side, avoiding social gatherings due to exhaustion and the fear of depressing her friends. "I feel responsible, like I could have done something to prevent this," she said, guilt evident in hervoice.

"I feel torn apart," Mrs. X's weight loss was a visible sign of her stress. "They suggest hospice, but we're scared it means giving up. We know this isn't the best place for him, but we can't decide," she confessed.

As time passed, it became clear that Mr. X's condition was beyond recovery. Another bout of pneumonia struck. "What can we do now?" she asked. We often talk about the Four Things that Matter Most (Byock, 2014).

"Thank you for loving me," she said, hervoice filled with love.

The case of Mr. and Mrs. X exemplifies the profound challenges faced by Chinese couples during terminal illness. Mrs. X's deep grief and sense of duty underscore the emotional burden borne by partners of the terminally ill. Her unwavering presence at her husband's side, coupled with her withdrawal from social life, reflects a strong sense of loyalty and commitment, yet also reveals her isolation and despair. The consideration of hospice care brings to light a prevalent misunderstanding in end-of-life (EoL) situations: many families perceive it as surrendering hope rather than as a compassionate approach to enhance quality of life through symptom management. This view often relegates hospice care to a last resort, overshadowing its value as a core aspect of patient-centered care.

Culturally, this case reflects the Confucian principles of family-centered decision-making. Mrs. X's comfort with family involvement in medical decisions and her feelings of guilt resonate with these cultural values. The scenario emphasizes the significance of relational autonomy in the Chinese setting, where familial bonds profoundly influence individual decision-making.

The narrative above also touches on the concept of "The Four Things that Matter Most," which suggests a focus on essential emotional communications at the end of life: expressions of love, forgiveness, gratitude, and farewell. In "The Four Things That Matter Most," Ira Byock delves into end-of-life care, emphasizing emotional healing and wholeness despite death's inevitability. Byock, a renowned figure in palliative care, leverages his vast experience to guide readers on the four vital messages that can bring a sense of closure and peace to relationships: "Please forgive me," "I forgive you," "Thank you," and "I love you." These simple yet profound statements serve as powerful tools for healing strained relationships, conveying deep emotions, and fostering reconciliation at life's end.

Scenario 2: What CanHealthcare Providers Do?

(This scenario is based on interviews with two clinical oncologists who have extensive experience in end-of-life care in China.) Healthcare providers are instrumental in delivering compassionate EoLC that respects the cultural values and family dynamics of Chinese cancer patients. Dr. KC (personal communication, May 15, 2022) emphasizes the importance of involving close family members in decision-making processes. He notes that understanding family dynamics and identifying caregiver stress are key to facilitating effective communication and shared decision-making. "Make sure you involve close family members of the patient," Dr. KC advises, "and be sensitive to family dynamics, identify carer stress, and invite key persons for decision making."

As families grapple with the transition from curative treatment to EoLC, providers must manage the emotional impact on patients and families. Dr. KC explains, "We will make sure they understand no more treatment does not mean neglect; in fact, more treatments may bring harm and is of little if no benefit." He stresses the importance of educating families on expected symptoms and disease trajectory, helping families understand that "the disease has its own natural course and is usually difficult to be picked up at its early stage."

Clinical oncologist LF (personal communication, May 15, 2022) echoes these sentiments, highlighting the burdens placed on families suddenly thrust into caregiving roles. "They have to perform a load of new duties… such as seeing multiple doctors or health professionals; information overload, new caring tasks etc.," says Dr. LF. He notes the importance of preparing caregivers for what lies ahead, including "gradual deterioration of the patient," and ensuring they know how to act in emergencies.

> "When breathing is becoming difficult, they have to call the ambulance," says Dr. LF, "and it is crucial for us healthcare providers to facilitate discussions with the patient about their will, last wishes, and advanced directives." Dr. LF underscores that these conversations must be conducted "tactfully with time, and rapport these essential." Observing family dynamics and cultural attitudes towards death and suffering is vital. He acknowledges that while family can be a source of comfort for the patient, if not handled correctly, it can also present challenges.

Involving a patient's family in EoLC, while respecting the patient's relational autonomy, requires a delicate balance. Healthcare providers must recognize the patient's role within their family and the influence of familial relationships on their decision-making. It is essential to engage in open, culturally sensitive dialogue that includes both the patient and their family members. This approach ensures that the patient's wishes are heard and considered alongside the family's input. Providers can facilitate family meetings that encourage transparent discussions about the patient's preferences, prognosis, and care options. These meetings can help align the family's expectations with the patient's desires, fostering a supportive environment for shared decision-making. Providers should offer resources and support to help families cope with the emotional burden of caregiving and bereavement. In so doing, healthcare providers can honor both the individual autonomy of the patient and the collective voice of their family, ultimately leading to more personalized and respectful EoLC.

Communicating Under Time Constraints

In real-world clinical settings, particularly in busy public hospitals in Hong Kong and mainland China, time is a limited and precious resource. Physicians and nurses often face pressure to manage multiple patients while still delivering compassionate, patient-centered care. This is especially challenging in emotionally sensitive contexts such as end-of-life communication, where quality conversations often require more time than the system allows.

To support clinicians in these fast-paced environments, time-efficient communication strategies can be adapted to maintain empathy, clarity, and effectiveness within a limited timeframe. Two practical approaches—**the 3-min consultationmodel** and **adapted ISBAR**—can help clinicians navigate this challenge.

The 3-Minute Consultation Model

This model encourages clinicians to structure conversations in three clear stages:

1. **Minute 1—Establishing Rapport and Setting Expectations**
   Begin with a warm greeting and orient the patient and/or family to the purpose of the conversation (e.g., discussing prognosis, options, or next steps). A brief empathetic statement can immediately signal care and openness.
2. **Minute 2—Communicating Key Information**
   Share essential medical facts in clear, non-technical language. Focus on one or two key messages (e.g., "The treatment is no longer effective) and avoid overwhelming the listener.
3. **Minute 3—Emotional Acknowledgment and Next Steps**
   Acknowledge the emotional impact of the information. Invite questions, offer supportive resources, and suggest follow-up actions. Even brief reassurance ("We are here for you") can have lasting effects.

This model is especially valuable during ward rounds or first-time palliative care discussions, providing a structured yet humane way to communicate efficiently.

ISBAR for End-of-Life Care

Originally designed for clinical handovers, **ISBAR** (Identify, Situation, Background, Assessment, Recommendation) can be adapted for sensitive EoL conversations among healthcare providers or during brief family discussions.

- **Identify**: Who is the patient, and who is involved in the conversation?
- **Situation**: What is the immediate concern (e.g., worsening condition, new symptoms)?
- **Background**: What is the patient's cancer stage, prior care plan, or wishes?
- **Assessment**: What is your clinical judgment or emotional insight at this point?
- **Recommendation**: What is the proposed next step—e.g., initiate family meeting, revise care goals, or consult palliative team?

By following a shared framework, interdisciplinary teams and family caregivers can align quickly, even under time constraints. To summarise, integrating time-efficient communication strategies does not imply reducing empathy or quality. Instead, these models provide **practical scaffolding** for clinicians to deliver culturally sensitive, clear, and supportive messages—even in busy oncology wards. Their use can enhance patient-centered care while reducing clinician stress and communication errors.

Conclusion

In conclusion, end-of-life care communication within the Chinese context requires a delicate interplay between medical realism and cultural empathy. The principles of filial piety and familial harmony are deeply embedded in the Chinese ethos, necessitating healthcare providers to approach EoLC with a culturally sensitive lens. By analyzing real-life scenarios and interviews, this chapter underscores the importance of engaging family members in the EoLC process while upholding the relational autonomy of patients. It is imperative that healthcare professionals are equipped with strategies that navigate the complexities of cultural expectations without compromising the dignity and individual desires of Chinese cancer patients. As we strive for a "good death," it is clear that culturally congruent care is not just a medical necessity but a moral imperative that honors the patient's life journey and provides solace to those they leave behind.

Discussion Prompts

1. What are the key cultural values that shape end-of-life (EoL) communication in Chinese cancer care, and how do they differ from Western practices?
2. How do Confucian concepts like filial piety and relational autonomy influence decision-making in EoLC?
3. What challenges do healthcare providers face when balancing transparency with respect for family-centered decision-making in the Chinese context?
4. In what ways does the case of Mr. and Mrs. X illustrate the emotional and cultural complexities of EoLC?
5. How can family meetings be used effectively to align patient wishes with family expectations in EoLC scenarios?

Reflection Questions

1. Reflect on a situation where you (or someone you know) had to make a medical decision for a family member. How were cultural or family values involved in that process?
2. How would you approach delivering EOL information to a patient whose family insists on withholding the diagnosis? What communication strategies would you use?
3. What does the concept of a "good death" mean in the context of your own cultural background? How does it compare with the values presented in this chapter?
4. How can healthcare systems better support both clinicians and families in navigating the emotional burden of EOL communication?
5. After reading this chapter, how would you revise your own approach to discussing palliative care and advanced directives with patients from diverse cultural backgrounds?

References

Bhadelia, A., Oldfield, L. E., Cruz, J. L., Singh, R., & Finkelstein, E. A. (2022). Identifying core domains to assess the "quality of death": A scoping review. *Journal of Pain and Symptom Management, 63*(4), e365–e386.

Bray, F., Laversanne, M., Sung, H., Ferlay, J., Siegel, R. L., Soerjomataram, I., & Jemal, A. (2024). Global cancer statistics 2022: GLOBOCAN estimates of incidence and mortality worldwide for 36 cancers in 185 countries. *CA: A Cancer Journal for Clinicians, 74*(3), 229–263.

Byock, I. (2014). *The four things that matter most: A book about living*. Simon and Schuster.

Chen, W., Zhang, L., Hu, M., & Hu, S. (2023). Use of health technology assessment in drug reimbursement decisions in China. *BMJ*, 381.

Cheng, Q., Duan, Y., Zheng, H., Xu, X., Khan, K., Xie, J., & Chen, Y. (2021). Knowledge, attitudes and preferences of palliative and end-of-life care among patients with cancer in mainland China: A cross-sectional study. *British Medical Journal Open, 11*(9), Article e051735.

Chung, R. Y. N., & Yeoh, E. K. (2019). Policy directions for end-of-life care in Hong Kong. In I. K. N. Chan, C. H. C. Fong, E. Y. Wong, V. W. Q. Lou, & C. L. W. Chan (Eds.), *The foundation of community-based end-of-life care in Hong Kong* (pp. 41–56). The Jockey Club End-of-Life Community Care Project.

Cong, Y. (2022). The dilemma and way out of hospice care in China. *Chinese Medical Journal, 102*(48), 3815–3818. https://doi.org/10.3760/cma.j.cn112137-20220803-01683

Egan, K. A., & Labyak, M. J. (2006). Hospice Palliative Care: A model for quality end-of-life care. *Textbook of Palliative Nursing*, 33.

Gong, X.-Q., & Bai, H.-N. (2022). Research on the policy diffusion of hospice care in Shanghai: Text analysis based on 56 hospice policies. *Chinese Journal of Health Policy, 15*(7), 30–37.

Hagerty, R. G., Butow, P. N., Ellis, P. M., Dimitry, S., & Tattersall, M. H. N. (2005). Communicating prognosis in cancer care: A systematic review of the literature. *Annals of Oncology, 16*(7), 1005–1053.

Hahne, J., Wang, X., Liu, R., Zhong, Y., Chen, X., Lui, X., Khoshnood, K., Li, X. (2022).Chinese physicians' perceptions of palliative care integration for advanced cancer patients: a qualitative analysis at a tertiary hospital in ChangshaChina*BMC Medical Ethics, 23*, 17.

Han, B., Zheng, R., Zeng, H., Wang, S., Sun, K., Chen, R., Li, L., Wei, W., & He, J. (2024). Cancer incidence and mortality in China, 2022. *Journal of the National Cancer Center, 4*(1), 47–53.

Hui, D., Nooruddin, Z., Didwaniya, N., Dev, R., De La Cruz, M., Kim, S. H., Kwon, J. H., Hutchins, R., Liem, C., & Bruera, E. (2014). Concepts and definitions for "actively dying," "end of life," "terminally ill," "terminal care," and "transition of care": A systematic review. *Journal of Pain and Symptom Management, 47*(1), 77–89.

Institute of Medicine. (2015). Dying in America: Improving quality and honoring individual preferences near the end of life.

Jeon, E. D., & Jing, J. (2023). A study of end-of-life care communication and decision-making in China by exploring filial piety and medical information concealment. *American Journal of Medical Humanities, 2*(1).

Leng, A., Maitland, E., Wang, S., Nicholas, S., Lan, K., & Wang, J. (2022). Preferences for end-of-life care among patients with terminal cancer in China. *JAMA Network Open, 5*(4), Article e228788.

Luk, J. K. H., Liu, A. N. C., Ng, W. C., Beh, S. L., & Chan, F. H. W. (2011). End-of-life care in Hong Kong. *Asian Journal of Gerontology and Geriatrics, 6*(2), 103–106.

Luta, X., Ottino, B., Hall, P., Bowden, J., Wee, B., Droney, J., Riley, J., & Marti, J. (2021). Evidence on the economic value of end-of-life and palliative care interventions: a narrative review of reviews. *BMC Palliative Care, 20*(1), 89.

Maubach, N., Batten, M., Jones, S., Chen, J., Scholz, B., Davis, A., Bromley, J., Burke, B., Tan, R., Hurwitz, M., Rodgers, H., & Mitchell, I. (2019). End-of-life care in an Australian acute hospital: A retrospective observational study. *Internal Medicine Journal, 49*(11), 1400–1405.

Miller, E. M., Porter, J. E., & Barbagallo, M. S. (2022). The experiences of health professionals, patients, and families with truth disclosure when breaking bad news in palliative care: A qualitative meta-synthesis. *Palliative & Supportive Care, 20*(3), 433–444.

PDQ Supportive and Palliative Care Editorial Board. (2024). Planning the transition to end-of-life care in advanced cancer (PDQ®): Health Professional Version. In *PDQ Cancer Information Summaries*. National Cancer Institute (US).

Pun, J. K. H., Cheung, K. M., Chow, J. C. H., & Chan, W. L. (2020). Chinese perspective on end-of-life communication: A systematic review. *BMJ Supportive & Palliative Care, 14*(e1), e30-e37.

Ricoeur, P. (1992). *Oneself as another*. University of Chicago Press.

Sleeman, K. E., de Brito, M., Etkind, S., Nkhoma, K., Guo, P., Higginson, I. J., Gomes, B., & Harding, R. (2019). The escalating global burden of serious health-related suffering: Projections to 2060 by world regions, age groups, and health conditions. *The Lancet. Global Health, 7*(7), e883–e892.

Walczak, A., Butow, P. N., Tattersall, M. H., Davidson, P. M., Young, J., Epstein, R. M., Costa, D. S. J., & Clayton, J. M. (2017). Encouraging early discussion of life expectancy and end-of-life care: a randomised controlled trial of a nurse-led communication support program for patients and caregivers. *International journal of nursing studies, 67,* 31–40.

Wang, H., Zhao, F., Wang, X., & Chen, X. (2018). To tell or not: The Chinese doctors' dilemma on disclosure of a cancer diagnosis to the patient. *Iranian Journal of Public Health, 47*(11), 1773–1774.

Wright, A. A., Keating, N. L., Balboni, T. A., Matulonis, U. A., Block, S. D., & Prigerson, H. G. (2010). Place of death: Correlations with quality of life of patients with cancer and predictors of bereaved caregivers' mental health. *Journal of Clinical Oncology, 28*(29), 4457–4464.

Yan, Y., Zhang, H., Gao, W., Liu, D., Endo, M., Deshpande, G. A., Uehara, Y., Watanabe, D., Yoshikawa, S., & Mizushima, A. (2020). Current awareness of palliative care in China. *The Lancet. Global Health, 8*(3), e333–e335.

Yee, H. H., Fong, B. Y., & Ng, T. K. (2020). Overview of palliative care service in Hong Kong. *Asia Pacific Journal of Health Management, 15*(2), 39–44.

Chapter 7
"How Much Time Do I Have?" Prognostication in Palliative Care from a Clinician's Perspective

Sunny Kong

Summary
This chapter explores prognostication from a Chinese palliative care physician's perspective. Time plays a crucial role in our lives, influencing the decisions we make. Patients and their families often seek answers to the challenging question of what the future holds. Prognostication involves estimating a patient's life expectancy (*"Fore-seeing"*) and communicating this information (*"Foretelling"*). It helps healthcare providers, patients, and families make important decisions, not just about medical treatment but also about other aspects of life. To be skilled at *"foretelling"*, it is essential to understand the cultural values of the people involved and address ethical concerns. The chapter presents various scenarios to illustrate the complexities of prognostication in the context of Chinese society, in which the importance of the relational self sometimes surpasses that of an individual. Ultimately, the question of "how much time do I have" goes beyond a simple countdown, reflecting a deeper desire for answers that go beyond the constraints of time.

Introduction

Palliative care physicians practising in acute hospital settings often encounter patients during the most challenging moments of their lives. Some patients are in the final stages of their journey, facing imminent mortality, while others have recently received the devastating news of a terminal diagnosis, such as cancer or organ failure. The question that frequently arises in these situations is, "How much time do I have?" This inquiry is often accompanied by profound emotional intensity, reflecting the

S. Kong (✉)
Department of Medicine, Hong Kong Buddhist Hospital, Hong Kong, China
e-mail: sunny.kong@ha.org.hk

J. Pun (ed.), *Teaching and Learning Oncology Communication*,
https://doi.org/10.1007/978-981-96-9474-7_7

inherent uncertainty of the future and the resulting apprehension and loss of control over one's individualistic and relational aspects.

Erik Cassel (1982) portrays suffering as not only a physical experience but also as a threat to the intricate social and psychological integrity of an individual. Failure to comprehend a patient's suffering may lead to unnecessary medical interventions that inadvertently become a source of additional suffering, ultimately resulting in a death stripped of dignity and a guilt-ridden family. Without proper prognostication, decision-making along the disease journey is akin to cruising through a stormy sea without any navigational tools. Blinded, hasty and rough decisions for medical treatment and personal issues are unlikely to adequately address suffering, if not worsen it.

The primary objective of palliative care is to enhance the well-being of patients and their families who are facing the challenges of life-threatening illnesses. It aims to prevent and alleviate suffering by promptly identifying, accurately assessing, and effectively treating physical, psychosocial, and spiritual problems. The scope of palliative care extends beyond the management of physical symptoms, encompassing a holistic approach to address various aspects of suffering. Therefore, palliative care clinicians need to be proficient in prognostication to guide patients and families in setting realistic expectations and meaningful goals for care.

However, within certain cultural contexts, disclosing prognostic information may be perceived as distressing. For instance, within Chinese society, there is often a reluctance to divulge unfavourable prognosis or even the mere diagnosis of a terminal illness to patients. Even when families consent to the disclosure of prognostic information, healthcare professionals often experience significant stress and difficulty in making predictions about survival. Patients and families expect clinicians to prognosticate in a manner that is simultaneously, yet impossibly, honest, accurate, and optimistic (Christakis, 1999). This raises moral and ethical questions regarding the practice of clinicians. Consequently, clinicians may become even more hesitant to engage in explicit discussions or document these prognoses.

Despite these challenges, prognostication remains both essential and unavoidable, serving the best interests of all parties involved. Palliative care clinicians should communicate prognosis in a manner that aligns with the needs of the patients. Ultimately, prognostication should be evidence-based, adaptable and patient-centred.

The aim of this chapter is, in its most modest scope, to examine the essence of prognostication and the cultural implications it carries from the perspective of a Hong Kong Chinese palliative care physician. By highlighting the obstacles encountered and ethical concerns through practical scenarios, this chapter seeks to provide insights into the complex nature of prognostication in palliative care within the Hong Kong Chinese cultural context.

Prognostication

Prognosis, a critical aspect of healthcare, is composed of two key elements: "*foreseeing*" and "*foretelling*" (Lamont & Christakis, 1999). "*Foreseeing*" refers to a clinician's cognitive prediction of a patient's illness trajectory. This prediction is based on a thorough understanding of the disease's natural course, the effects of various treatment options on survival, and individual patient factors such as comorbidities and functional status. This process involves both intuitive predictions by clinicians and actuarial estimations that compute probabilities by integrating relevant parameters into various models. While there have been substantial advancements in developing robust prognostic models using big data and machine learning techniques (Schaar & Hemingway, 2019), accurately predicting a patient's survival remains a significant challenge. This is particularly true when it comes to determining the appropriate time to acknowledge that a patient is nearing the end of life. The intricacies involved in "*foreseeing*" warrant a detailed discussion of their own.

On the other hand, "*foretelling*" pertains to the conveyance of prognostic information to patients and their significant others. It is crucial to ensure that patients and their families have a comprehensive understanding of the patient's health status and what the future may hold. Our capacity to effectively communicate with patients and their families is equally important to "*foreseeing*." By ensuring they have a comprehensive understanding of what lies ahead, we can translate this knowledge into meaningful outcomes that truly benefit them, providing the support they need during challenging times.

Prognostication is a multistep process (Hui et al., 2021). It begins with clinicians making predictions and acknowledging the need for discussing prognostic information (prognostic formulation). Subsequently, clinicians engage in discussions about prognosis after clarifying the patients' interest (prognostic disclosure). For patients to effectively utilise prognostic information, they must comprehend the predictions provided (prognostic awareness), emotionally process these expectations (prognostic acceptance), and make personal and healthcare plans based on the prognosis (prognosis-based decision-making).

The proposed conceptual framework highlights five patient categories depending on their desire for prognostic information, awareness, and acceptance. These groups are Avoidance ("*I don't want to know*"), Discordant ("*I never wanted to know*"), Anxious ("*I don't know what's happening*"), Concerned ("*I don't like this*"), Acceptance ("*I know how to plan ahead*"). It is crucial to underscore that prognostication is not a singular, linear process. By delineating the patient's cognitive and emotional state within the continuum of prognostication, healthcare professionals can provide customised interventions to enhance decision-making abilities and ultimately enhance patient outcomes. Nonetheless, Hui (2021) has highlighted the delicate nature of these discussions and raised concerns regarding the potential adverse consequences that may arise if the conversations are inappropriately conducted.

Building on this, it is important to note that communication, a key aspect of prognostication, is heavily influenced by culture. Understanding cultural norms and value systems can improve the quality of care by healthcare professionals through sensitive and individualised communication (Gilligan, 2018). Hong Kong culture, with its colonial history, is a unique blend of Western and Chinese influences that incorporates elements from both. At the same time, most Hong Kong Chinese maintain strong ties to their Chinese roots, such as the traditional values of filial piety and the priority of the family, which continue to shape the social fabric of Hong Kong society. It is important to note that Hong Kong's Chinese culture is not solely defined by Western or Chinese values but rather a fusion and adaptation of these diverse elements. The fusion and adaptation challenge the communication skills and the ethical balance of healthcare professionals working in the locality.

Cultural Considerations

Culture is a multifaceted concept that encompasses traditions, beliefs, values, norms, and meanings that are collectively embraced, to differing extents, by individuals within a community. Culture pertains to the shared perceptions and standards that form the acquired frameworks of significance within a specific community. In addition, culture plays a role in shaping the perceived importance of responsibilities, obligations, and familial interdependence, as well as the relative involvement of the patient compared to other parties in medical decision-making. In turn, culture influences the perceived level of potential harm associated with the decision-making process (Ting-Toomey & Chung, 2012).

Disparities exist in cultural perspectives. Asian cultures have traditionally tended to discourage truth-telling and favour decision-making processes centred around the family unit. Social expectations and emotions are often implied rather than explicitly expressed. Direct communication may be perceived as impolite, leading individuals to convey their true intentions more subtly and anticipate others to discern their emotions and respond accordingly (Mori, 2023). In the context of Chinese society, it was traditionally believed to be inappropriate to discuss the diagnosis and prognosis with terminally ill patients openly. This belief stems from the notion that such discussions about death are associated with misfortune and disrupt inner harmony.

From our clinical experience, the opinions of the patient's family sometimes carry as much, if not more, weight than those of the patient. Consequently, doctors rarely make decisions solely in consultation with their patients. The pressure exerted by family members to withhold information from the patient further complicates the challenges associated with providing appropriate palliative care. Understandably, clinicians may fear being blamed and provoking anger from both the patient and their family when delivering the news of an unfavourable prognosis.

Within the Chinese medical community, there is also a prevailing perception that the primary objective of medicine is to sustain life at all costs. In this context, palliative care and acceptance of death are viewed as a failure of medicine. While healthcare professionals in China generally acknowledge the need for palliative care for terminally ill patients, they often refrain from directly providing this care themselves because of the challenge of dealing with the concept of death (Stocklassa et al., 2021). Receiving palliative care services is often interpreted as merely waiting for the patient to die or as a form of masked euthanasia.

Contrarily, terminally ill cancer patients in China have a preference for being informed about their diagnosis and prognosis, as it allows them to prepare for the inevitability of death. The primary objective of palliative care is to ensure a dignified and satisfactory end-of-life experience, which can vary based on individual interpretations. It is essential to identify the unique values and expectations of patients regarding a "good death" to provide quality palliative care.

Additionally, considering the specific cultural context of cancer patients in China is crucial. While it is common for individuals in China to withhold information about terminal illness from their family members, they often desire to be informed if they are facing a similar situation (Stocklassa et al., 2021). Therefore, understanding the Chinese cultural beliefs surrounding disclosure and death would be essential in handling the delicate conversation of prognosis discussion.

Challenges in the Chinese Context

Besides cultural considerations, clinicians face challenges that test their communication skills and ethical judgement, as they must strike a delicate balance between instilling hope and setting achievable goals. Engaging in emotionally charged conversations requires addressing several crucial questions: identifying who the decision-maker is, ensuring that they possess sufficient information to make informed choices, and determining the desired level of disclosure for both the patient and their family. In the context of Chinese culture, it is essential to consider how patients and families perceive their roles in decision-making regarding care plans. Additionally, handling situations where patients explicitly request to be kept unaware of critical information requires careful understanding and navigation. The following scenarios (modified from real-life examples to ensure anonymity) serve as illustrations of common yet complex situations where cultural norms and ethical considerations intersect.

Scenario 1: When the Family Asks not to disclose to the Patient

In the clinic, Mrs A arrived in a wheelchair, accompanied by her daughters. One of them gently pushed the wheelchair as they entered the consultation room. As I reviewed the previous clinical notes on the computer, it became evident that Mrs H was diagnosed with metastatic lung cancer.

"Good Morning, Mrs H! How Are You Feeling Today?" I Greeted Her with a Smile.

"It feels like having cancer!" Mrs A responded, displaying a hint of wit in her smile.

Curious About Her Statement, I Inquired Further, "and What Do You Mean by that?"

With a subtle gesture, one of Mrs A's daughters moved her lips, silently indicating that her mother was unaware of the metastasis. She shook her head, signalling me not to disclose this information to Mrs A.

Chinese patients have demonstrated a desire to receive information about their diagnosis and prognosis directly, rather than relying on their family members for communication. While research suggests that Chinese patients generally appreciate being informed about their end-of-life care (Lou et al., 2023; Sun et al., 2015), our clinical experience indicates that Chinese family members tend to avoid disclosing the truth to patients. This is often motivated by the principle of nonmaleficence (Chan, 2011). Family members and patients in Chinese culture have a strong interdependence. Patients rely on their family members for emotional support and decision-making. The support and acceptance of caregivers are seen as crucial personal resources that can positively impact the psychosocial well-being of Chinese patients. Consequently, family members still hold significant influence in determining whether patients should be informed of the truth. If they believe that disclosing the diagnosis or prognosis would be harmful to the patient, they may object to the disclosure and convince healthcare professionals to withhold the truth.

However, nonmaleficence hardly justifies nondisclosure, and it can be detrimental to palliative care patients. At some point, most of our patients may come to terms with the fact that their life will come to an end, whether it be sooner or later. However, by denying patients the opportunity to comprehend the trajectory of their illness and anticipate the dying process, patients are left in a state of uncertainty and anxiety (Tse et al., 2003). Tragedies can happen overnight: the loss of cognitive function due to brain metastasis resulting in the loss of self and identity; the sudden loss of mobility from spinal cord compression due to bone metastasis, coupled with the subsequent loss of freedom and ability for self-care. Nothing seems so feared as the loss of self-determination and the erosion of dignity. To have a choice is to have some control, even a choice to do nothing. It is this lack of anticipation regarding the dying process and the duration before death occurs that causes immense distress for our patients. It is through an awareness of the dying process that patients can better cope with the challenges they face.

Scenario 2: When the Patient Asks not to disclose to the Family

Mr. B suffered from metastatic nasopharyngeal cancer, enduring the excruciating pain caused by bone metastasis. His appetite deteriorated and cachexia further weakened his body. Aware of his limited time left, Mr. B understood the gravity of his situation.

His children, residing in the Overseas, were only informed about his condition while he underwent palliative chemotherapy.

"Have you Ever Considered Telling Them?" I Asked, Curious About His Perspective.

With a sombre expression, Mr. B replied, "There's nothing they can do to help. I am dying. I would rather have them remember me as the robust father I once was, rather than burdening them with this horrendous journey. Once I am gone, they will moan, but they need not endure this painful process alongside me."

It may not be possible to change someone's perspective. However, patients' self-perceived burden on the family may hinder their children from fulfilling their obligations of filial piety, leading to lasting regrets. As the disease advances, patients may lose the ability to make decisions for themselves. If the family is not adequately informed about the prognosis, they may make decisions that do not align with the patient's preferences. It is important to understand why patients choose not to disclose their prognosis and consider alternatives, such as finding common ground or determining an appropriate time for the patient to share their prognosis with their family.

Scenario 3: Mutual Pretence

Miss C, a university student, suffered from metastaticcancer of unknown origin. Her parents' divorce shortly after her birth left her to be raised by her young mother, their lives intricately intertwined in a symbiotic dance of interdependence. As her organs began to fail, Miss C became frail and confined to her bed, her body swollen with oedema and her complexion marred by a deep jaundice. It was during this time that we first encountered her, receiving supportive transfusions and antibiotics infusion.

"My mother is my pillar of strength," Miss C confided, her voiceVoice filled with determination. "I must hold onto hopeHope for her sake. I am willing to endure the pain of chemotherapyChemotherapy and clinical trials if it means prolonging my life. The thought of leaving my mother behind is unbearable." Curiosity compelled us to ask, "Have you shared your feelings about the treatments with your mother?" A shadow of hesitation crossed Miss C's face. "No," she admitted, her voiceVoice barely above a whisper. "I couldn't bear to burden her with my desire to give up. I have chosen to keep my struggles hidden, to maintain an illusion of hopeHope."

As we engaged in conversation, Mrs C, Miss C's mother, arrived at the ward during visiting hours. Sensing her distress, we introduced ourselves as the palliative care team, and she beckoned us to speak with her. Tears streamed down her face as she pleaded, "Can you help my daughter?" We paused for a moment, recognising the anguish of a parent faced with the impending loss of her child. "How can we help?" we asked, acknowledging the desperate yearning for a cure that was, unfortunately, nearly impossible to attain. Mrs C's sobs intensified, her words punctuated by gasps for air. "I can't bear to see her suffer any longer," she managed to say. "I have felt her pain and witnessed her suffering throughout the treatments. I want to tell her that it's okay to let go, but the words won't escape my lips." The weight of her emotions mirrored the pain I could only imagine as a parent myself. "I must remain strong and hopeful because that is what she has done. She wants to live."

Both mother and daughter, each other's rock, were engaged in a silent pact of hope against the somewhat inevitable. This unspoken agreement, a poignant example of what Glaser and Strauss describe as the "ritual drama of mutual pretence," reveals the complex dynamic at play when confronting terminal illness (Glaser & Strauss, 2017). In such scenarios, patients, families, and healthcare providers often participate in a delicate charade, acting as if the progression towards death is not happening. This mutual pretence may serve as a coping mechanism, potentially easing immediate distress but also filtering the information shared, based on what doctors and families believe the patient should know. By selectively disclosing information, we risk eroding trust and damaging the very relationships we aim to protect. It raises profound ethical questions about autonomy and the right to make informed decisions about one's own life.

However unique our individuality, we live within cultural and familial contexts that involve obligations, duties, relationships, and interdependence. In many cases, especially in Chinese society, patients willingly consider how their decisions will affect their valued relationships and seek advice from family members or other important people in their lives. Cultural and interpersonal factors can influence the importance patients place on these considerations during their decision-making processes. Such considerations, when not coerced, can embody a legitimate expression of autonomy.

In healthcare, this concept of autonomy extends beyond the individual to encompass relational autonomy-a recognition of the interconnectedness of our choices (Gómez-Vírseda et al., 2020; Ho, 2008). Yet, apart from this relational aspect, there exists a phenomenon known as "necessary collusion" (Helft, 2005) or, more precisely, "voluntary diminished autonomy" (Cherny, 2012). This occurs when patients, wary of the potential harm from an overload of medical information or the weight of decision-making, opt for a less direct role in their care (Liang et al., 2022). They may prefer to entrust medical decisions to loved ones or healthcare professionals, aligning with a broader desire for guidance and support.

Understanding and respecting a patient's autonomy, therefore, is not a one-size-fits-all approach. It necessitates a nuanced appreciation of the patient's desired level of involvement and information disclosure (Gómez-Vírseda et al., 2020). Overzealous transparency or unwarranted candour, when not sought by the patient, can be perceived as an "assault of truth" (Buttow et al., 1997), infringing upon the patient's right to navigate their healthcare journey on their terms.

Fear of Death as a Worldwide Phenomenon

Cultural factors influence health perceptions and behaviours, yet they do not solely dictate patient preferences in healthcare (Rice, 2023; Sheeran, 2023). The relationship between culture and patient autonomy is complex; neither cultural background nor affiliation accurately predicts patient preferences regarding the amount of information they desire about their illness and prognosis, or their desired level of involvement in decision-making (Kolmes et al., 2024; Scharf et al., 2021). For instance, in Western contexts, an oversimplified view may lead to excessive disclosure to patients who might prefer less, while in non-Western settings, it could result in insufficient information for those who seek a more active role in their care decisions. Recognizing that communication and decision-making preferences are not inherently tied to culture is crucial. Preferences vary among individuals, and assumptions should not be made based on cultural stereotypes or family input alone. Each patient's preferences must be individually explored, and there is no substitute for this personalised approach.

An individual may rationally wish to be informed of bad news while emotionally not wanting to hear it. Unfortunately, modern medicine increasingly forces us to make choices and take charge of our medical care, even when some of us prefer passivity. The apprehension towards death and the societal reluctance to openly discuss death and the dying process are not confined to specific cultures but rather a socio-psychological phenomenon which is becoming more segregated, with death heavily regulated and institutionalised (Tse et al., 2003). The "wild death" (Callahan, 2000) of technological medicine since the nineteenth century has made the course of death highly uncertain, bringing a type of death that gets the better of us, occurs at an undesired time, and often much later than it should have happened. This decline in health leaves us isolated and degraded, removed from the fitting and full presence in the life of the community. Death has evolved from a natural phenomenon to an alien and fearful event. The false narrative of medical cure comes at a great cost to the family who must continue living on with the knowledge that more truthful communication of prognosis could have changed the way patients lived at the end of life.

Compassion surpasses empathy as it recognizes and comprehends suffering, propels us to take action, and actively seeks voluntary acts of kindness. It is through compassion that we can transition from merely observing suffering to understanding the patient's needs within the context of their life, seeking assistance to meet those needs for both the patient and their family, and ultimately providing solutions. This is the essence of prognostication in palliative care.

Conclusion

Prognostication plays a crucial role in palliative care, allowing healthcare professionals to guide patients and their families through the challenges of life-threatening illnesses. However, within the cultural context of Hong Kong Chinese society, some unique considerations and challenges impact the communication and disclosure of prognostic information. The fusion of Western and Chinese influences, along with traditional values and beliefs, shapes the expectations and preferences of patients and their families regarding prognosis discussions.

Cultural norms in Hong Kong Chinese society often discourage direct and explicit communication about terminal illnesses, emphasising the importance of family unity and harmony. Clinicians must navigate these cultural sensitivities while providing accurate and meaningful prognostic information. Additionally, the role of family members in decision-making further complicates the process, as their opinions often hold significant influence.

The delicate nature of prognosis discussions highlights the need for healthcare professionals to possess strong communication skills, cultural competence, and ethical judgement. Customised interventions and a patient-centred approach are essential to meet the diverse needs and preferences of individuals within the continuum of prognostication.

By understanding the cultural nuances and balancing the ethical considerations, healthcare professionals can enhance the quality of care and support provided to patients and their families. Open and sensitive communication, tailored to individual preferences, can help patients make informed decisions, prepare for the future, and experience a dignified end-of-life journey. In this sense, the question of "How much time do I have" often transcends mere temporal considerations. It revolves around the actions that patients and their loved ones can undertake before the patient departs from this earthly world, ensuring the fulfilment of what truly holds significance in their lives.

Discussion Prompts

1. How do cultural norms in Hong Kong and broader Chinese society influence decisions about disclosing prognostic information to patients and families?
2. What are the key challenges in balancing honesty, empathy, and optimism when engaging in prognostic communication?
3. How do the concepts of relational autonomy and "voluntary diminished autonomy" complicate discussions of truth-telling in palliative care?
4. What ethical dilemmas arise when family members request non-disclosure of a terminal prognosis to the patient—or vice versa?
5. In what ways can clinicians navigate "mutual pretence" between patients and families, and what are the potential risks or benefits of this approach?

Reflection Questions

1. Reflect on the five patient categories related to prognostic awareness presented in the chapter. Where do you see yourself—or a loved one—falling within this spectrum, and why?
2. Have you ever experienced or witnessed a situation where medical information was intentionally withheld? What were the consequences of that decision?
3. How would you personally approach a situation where a patient does not want to disclose their prognosis to family members? What factors would guide your response?

4. In your own cultural background or personal values, what does a "good death" look like? How does that compare to the views expressed in this chapter?
5. What strategies from this chapter could you apply to improve your communication skills in delivering sensitive or emotionally charged information?

References

Buttow, N., Dunn, S., & Tattersall, H. N. (1997). Denial, misinformation, and the "assault of truth." In R. K. Portenoy & E. Bruera (Eds.), *Topics in palliative care* (Vol. 1, pp. 263–278). Oxford University Press.

Callahan, D. (2000). *The troubled dream of life: In search of a peaceful death.* Georgetown University Press.

Cassel, E. J. (1982). The nature of suffering and the goals of medicine. *New England Journal of Medicine, 306*(11), 639–645. https://doi.org/10.1056/NEJM198203183061104

Chan, W. C. (2011). Being aware of the prognosis: How does it relate to palliative care patients' anxiety and communication difficulty with family members in the Hong Kong Chinese context? *Journal of Palliative Medicine, 14*, 997–1003.

Cherny, N. I. (2012). Controversies in oncologist-patient communication: A nuanced approach to autonomy, culture, and paternalism. *Oncology, 26*(1), 37.

Christakis, N. A. (1999). Prognostication and bioethics. *Daedalus, 128*(4), 197–214.

Gilligan, T., Bohlke, K., & Baile, W. F. (2018). Patient-clinician communication: American Society of Clinical Oncology Consensus Guideline summary. *Journal of Oncology Practice, 14*, 42–46.

Glaser, B. G., & Strauss, A. L. (2017). *Awareness of dying.* Routledge.

Gómez-Vírseda, C., de Maeseneer, Y., & Gastmans, C. (2020). Relational autonomy in end-of-life care ethics: A contextualized approach to real-life complexities. *BMC Medical Ethics, 21*, 50.

Helft, P. R. (2005). Necessary collusion: Prognostic communication with advanced cancer patients. *Journal of Clinical Oncology, 23*(13), 3146–3150.

Ho, A. (2008). Relational autonomy or undue pressure? Family's role in medical decision-making. *Scandinavian Journal of Caring Sciences, 22*(1), 128–135.

Hui, D., Mo, L., & Paiva, C. E. (2021). The importance of prognostication: Impact of prognostic predictions, disclosures, awareness, and acceptance on patient outcomes. *Current Treatment Options in Oncology, 22*(2), 12.

Kolmes, S., Ha, C., & Potter, J. (2024). Responding to cultural limitations on patient autonomy: A clinical ethics case study. *HEC Forum, 36*, 99–109.

Lamont, E. B., & Christakis, N. A. (1999). Some elements of prognosis in terminal cancer. *Oncology, 13*(8), 1165–1180.

Liang, Z., Xu, M., Liu, G., et al. (2022). Patient-centered care and patient autonomy: Doctors' views in Chinese hospitals. *BMC Medical Ethics, 23*, 38.

Lou, Y., Liu, J., & Carr, D. (2023). To tell or not: Chinese older adults' preferences for disclosing or concealing serious illness diagnoses. *The Gerontologist, 63*(6), 1049–1059.

Mori, M., Lin, C. P., Cheng, S. Y., Suh, S. Y., Takenouchi, S., Ng, R., Chan, H., Kim, S. H., Chen, P. J., Yuen, K. K., Fujimori, M., Yamaguchi, T., Hamano, J., Kizawa, Y., Morita, T., & Martina, D. (2023). Communication in cancer care in Asia: A narrative review. *JCO Global Oncology, 9*, e2200266.

Rice, Z. S., & Liamputtong, P. (2023). Cultural determinants of health, cross-cultural research and global public health. In P. Liamputtong (Ed.), *Handbook of social sciences and global public health.* Springer.

Scharf, A., Voigt, L., Vardhana, S., Matsoukas, K., Wall, L. M., Arevalo, M., & Diamond, L. C. (2021). What should clinicians do when a patient's autonomy undermines her being treated equitably? *AMA Journal of Ethics, 23*(2), e97–e108.

Schaar, M. van, & Hemingway, H. (2019). Machine learning in prognosis research. *Prognosis Research in Health Care*, 328–342.

Sheeran, N., Jones, L., Pines, R., Jin, B., Pamoso, A., Eigeland, J., & Benedetti, M. (2023). How culture influences patient preferences for patient-centered care with their doctors. *Journal of Communication in Healthcare, 16*(2), 186–196.

Stocklassa, S., Zhang, S., Mason, S., & Elsner, F. (2021). Cultural implications for disclosure of diagnosis and prognosis toward terminally ill cancer patients in China: A literature review. *Palliative and Supportive Care, 20*, 283–289.

Sun, W., Wang, Z., Fang, S., & Li, M. (2015). Factors influencing the attitudes of Chinese cancer patients and their families toward the disclosure of a cancer diagnosis. *Journal of Cancer Education, 30*, 20–25.

Ting-Toomey, S., & Chung, L. C. (2012). Understanding intercultural communication (2nd ed.). Oxford University Press.

Tse, C. Y., Chong, A., & Fok, S. Y. (2003). Breaking bad news: A Chinese perspective. *Palliative Medicine, 17*, 339–343.

Chapter 8
Specific Roles of Family Members in Oncology Communication in Chinese Setting from a Clinician Perspective

Tsz Yeung Kam

Introduction

Effective communication is essential for high-quality oncology care, particularly within Chinese families, where patients often depend on shared decision-making with their close relatives. This chapter examines three case studies—Mr. C, Miss Y and Mr. W—all diagnosed with metastatic stage four lung cancer. These cases illustrate the practical aspects of oncology communication, emphasizing the vital role family members play in disclosing diagnoses, discussing treatment options, and planning advanced care in end-of-life situations. Through these journeys, we will analyze the complexities of these issues and the management of family involvement, particularly in the context of Chinese Communities.

Case of Mr. C—breaking Bad News

Mr. C was diagnosed with metastatic stage four lung cancer in 2015 at the age of 60. His diagnosis followed a series of investigations, including computed tomography (CT), positron emission tomography (PET)-CT, and a CT-guided lung biopsy. It was confirmed that Mr. C had EGFR (epidermal growth factor receptor) mutated non-small cell lung cancer (NSCLC), with metastases to the pleura and bones. While a diagnosis of stage four lung cancer typically carries a poor prognosis, advancements in cancer treatment, particularly EGFR targeted therapies, have significantly improved survival rates in recent years. For patients with EGFR mutations like Mr. C, the median survival with appropriate treatment is expected to be around 3 to 4 years.

T. Y. Kam (✉)
Hong Kong, China
e-mail: kty231@ha.org.hk

J. Pun (ed.), *Teaching and Learning Oncology Communication*,
https://doi.org/10.1007/978-981-96-9474-7_8

Mr. C has two sons and a daughter, all in their thirties, who work and live separately from him. Mr. C works as a school janitor and resides with his wife in Kowloon. Mr. C attended the oncology clinic accompanied by his two sons once the investigation results were available.

Delivery of Bad News

Importance of Effectively Breaking Bad News

Breaking bad news to oncology patients is a pivotal moment that significantly influences the quality of care. Bad news is defined as any news that adversely and seriously affects an individual's view of his or her future. The process of delivering bad news involves several crucial components, including understanding the patient's medical condition, evaluating the patient's attitudes, wishes, and needs, and addressing the emotional responses of both the patient and their family.

Good patient-centered communication fosters a supportive environment that enhances various outcomes. It leads to better medication adherence, improved pain management, and higher levels of patient satisfaction. Additionally, effective communication cultivates increased mutual trust between patients and healthcare providers, reduces psychological distress, and enhances coping mechanisms. By prioritizing effective communication, healthcare providers can help patients and their families navigate the challenges associated with a cancer diagnosis.

Role of Family in Breaking Bad News—Chinese Perspective

Family relationships and their involvement are critical external factors that greatly influence the decision-making process in oncology communication. In the context of Chinese culture, the role of the family assumes particularly significant importance. Research conducted in Hunan has shown that medical professionals frequently inform family members about a cancer diagnosis prior to discussing it with the patient, especially when the family expresses a desire to shield the patient from this distressing information. Three main reasons have emerged to explain this practice: first, there is a pervasive concern that many patients may lack the emotional resilience necessary to cope with bad news; second, healthcare providers often harbor fears of potential legal or interpersonal conflicts with family members; and third, there exists a fundamental ethical dilemma between respecting the patient's right to be informed about their health condition and honoring the family's interest in protecting the patient from emotional distress.

Anecdotal evidence gathered from Chinese patients residing in Western countries further underscores the strong objections expressed by family members regarding the idea of informing the patient about their diagnosis or prognosis. In Hong Kong, where the majority of the population is ethnically Chinese, Fielding reported that doctors disclosed the cancer diagnosis to only 68% of 133 terminal cancer patients. Even more concerning, the rate of prognostic disclosure was found to be just 38%. Despite the fact that 92% of doctors stated that they would disclose a diagnosis in principle, the reality of their practices often did not align with these intentions. A comprehensive survey conducted in 1996 revealed that a striking 95% of 1,136 individuals wanted to receive information about their health conditions, even if the news was unfavorable. This disparity highlights a significant gap between the preferences of family members and the individual desires of patients regarding information disclosure.

Moreover, cross-cultural differences regarding communication preferences have become increasingly apparent. In various Asian studies, it has been found that fewer than 30% of patients expressed a desire to discuss their life expectancy, while approximately 60% of patients in Western studies preferred to engage in such discussions. In Japan, a noteworthy 78% of patients indicated that they wished to receive bad news in the presence of family members. In contrast, this preference was significantly lower in other countries; only 40% of patients in Ireland, 53–57% in Australia, and 61% in Portugal expressed a desire to have family members present. Interestingly, a substantial 81% of patients in the United States preferred to receive bad news without anyone else present, including family members.

Essence of Breaking a "Good" Bad News

When it comes to delivering bad news, providing emotional support and employing appropriate manners are essential components of effective communication. It is crucial to express genuine empathy, speak in a gentle and soothing manner, and communicate in a way that inspires hope. Physical contact, such as touching or hugging, should generally be avoided unless the patient explicitly initiates such interactions. Utilizing supportive language can significantly alleviate the emotional distress experienced by the patient, and it is vital to allow the patient the space to express their feelings while simultaneously offering reassurance. Furthermore, encouraging patients to ask questions is an indispensable aspect of the communication process, as it fosters a sense of involvement and empowerment.

According to Maiko Fujimori et al., several key settings can enhance the effectiveness of breaking bad news. These settings include ensuring a high degree of privacy, conducting face-to-face consultations, and providing undivided attention to the patient during the conversation. It was showed that younger patients, female patients, and those with higher levels of education consistently express a strong desire for detailed information as well as emotional support during these difficult discussions. This highlights the need for healthcare providers to be particularly attentive to the specific needs and preferences of different patient groups when navigating the sensitive terrain of delivering bad news.

Breaking Bad News to Mr. C—Practical Aspect

In addressing Mr. C's condition, our oncologist typically begins the conversation by clarifying the understanding of his medical situation for both the patient and his family members. We take a methodical approach, slowly reiterating the initial investigations conducted by our specialists prior to the consultation. This practice demonstrates to Mr. C and his family that we have thoroughly reviewed all available information, which helps to build rapport between the patient and the clinician. Additionally, it serves to double-check their understanding of his underlying condition before we discuss treatment options.

For instance, in Mr. C's case, we would state, "We understand that you have been experiencing cough and shortness of breath for a couple of months. Your medical colleagues have referred you for a series of investigations, including imaging scans such as a CT scan and a PET scan. Following these scans, a biopsy was performed, which confirmed the presence of abnormal cells. The biopsy results indicated that these malignant cells originated from the lung and have spread to other organs, such as the bones. We are here today to discuss the best way to manage your condition moving forward."

It will be complemented with basic history taking and physical examination to assess the different aspects of the patient, including the physical, psychological and social functioning which contribute to the whole picture of the patient before discussing the available treatment and the overall care plan of the patient.

Discussion of Treatment Options with Mr's C Family

The discussion surrounding treatment options can be particularly sensitive, as it often requires confirming specific details that may evoke strong emotional responses. Furthermore, in public healthcare settings, if treatment options are not fully subsidized by the government, this can lead to potential conflicts between family members and the patient.

In practice, Chinese patients, especially when accompanied by family members such as children, often exhibit reluctance to engage in conversations about their prognosis, particularly if the patient is feeling unwell. Family members may attempt to withhold the diagnosis from the patient, fearing that this information could negatively impact their emotional well-being, making discussion of treatment options difficult.

In general, we have to be honest to give all available treatment options for the disease even with the fact that some of the options may not be affordable, as giving available options are the one of the best way to establish the rapport between the clinician and the family. And if there is no immediate urgency to start oncological treatment, most of the occasion a follow up appointment may be considered such that the patient and the family would have a chance to discuss with the patient individually as patient and family may feel pressured if they have to make a decision in the first consultation in front of the physician.

Moreover, with the advancements in oncological treatments, it becomes increasingly challenging to provide a precise prognosis. In Mr. C's case, while the median survival rate for patients with his condition is generally estimated at about 3 to 4 years, the actual trajectory of the disease can vary significantly. Experienced oncologists are cautious about making definitive predictions, especially at the initial diagnosis stage when multiple lines of treatment may be available in the future.

When patients inquire about their prognosis, our approach is usually to communicate openly and honestly. We emphasize the variability in individual responses to systemic treatments, which can lead to different outcomes. This uncertainty necessitates a careful and compassionate approach to discussions about prognosis, ensuring that patients are informed without being overwhelmed.

What if—Doctor, I Do not Want to Disclose the Diagnosis to My Father /Mother!

Case of Miss C

Miss C is an 83 year old lady with past medical history of hypertension, diabetes mellitus and ischemic heart disease. She is activity of daily living (ADL) partially dependent. She lives with her daughter and maid in a private housing, and a strong family support from her daughter and her three sons who are living apart. She is mainly taken care by the maid daytime when her daughter is working.

A diagnosis of metastatic lung cancer is made by a finding of chest X ray showing right pleural effusion, which subsequently pleural tapping was performed and revealed non-small-cell lung cancer. Genetic profiling was performed and revealed no druggable driver mutations. As patient ECOG is 3, she is physically not fit to receive any kind of palliative chemotherapy.

She attended the oncology clinic with her daughter. While we are going to see the patient and her daughter, her daughter entered the consultant room first, and requested the oncologist not to disclose the diagnosis to the patient, worrying that it would negatively impact the emotional status of the patient which may further worsened the clinical condition. On further discussion, the family expressed strong wish of palliative care and refused any active oncologist treatment, they are in the hope of minimize the impact of the diagnosis to the patient psychological well-being.

ARCHES Framework

The ARCHES framework is particularly useful in situations where families request non-disclosure of a diagnosis to the patient. This strategy is designed to precede the SPIKES protocol, which is commonly used for delivering bad news. ARCHES helps healthcare providers navigate the delicate balance between respecting family wishes and ensuring that the patient's right to know is upheld.

ARCHES stands for:

- **Acknowledgements**: Recognize the family's concerns and their desire to protect the patient. This acknowledgment is crucial in building trust and rapport. It is particularly import in Chinese family as family
- **Respect**: Show respect for the family's perspective and their motivations. Understanding that their intentions often stem from a place of love and concern is vital for effective communication.
- **Clarify**: Clarify any misunderstandings or misperceptions that may exist regarding the diagnosis or treatment options. This step is essential to ensure that everyone involved has a clear and accurate understanding of the situation.
- **Help**: Offer assistance in navigating the complex emotions that arise during these discussions. This may include providing emotional support to both the patient and the family, as well as facilitating conversations about treatment pathways.
- **Engage**: Actively involve both the patient and the family in the decision-making process. This engagement fosters a sense of collaboration and shared responsibility in managing the patient's care.

In discussions related to cancer diagnoses, healthcare providers often adopt specific language to facilitate better understanding and emotional comfort for both patients and their families. For instance, using terms like "tumors" instead of "cancer" can soften the impact of the diagnosis. Similarly, we might refer to "spread to another organ" rather than "metastasis" to make the medical terminology less daunting. Instead of labelling a condition as "incurable," we might frame it as "aiming for disease control and prevention of further progression." This approach emphasizes a proactive strategy, focusing on management rather than despair.

Upholding Confidentiality and Patient Rights

Throughout this process, it is essential to maintain the patient's confidentiality and uphold their right to knowledge. While respecting the family's wishes is important, it should not come at the expense of the patient's autonomy. The ARCHES framework encourages open dialogue that respects the family's concerns while simultaneously ensuring that the patient is informed about their health status and treatment options. This balanced approach not only empowers patients but also strengthens the overall therapeutic alliance between healthcare providers, patients, and families.

Communication with Miss C's Family

Our oncologist starts with "We as doctors understand the family concern of letting Miss C knowing the diagnosis of lung cancer, and it is especially challenging if letting an elderly knowing this. Your act is not unusual and actually many other families we saw shared similar thought. We can feel that you love and care Miss C very much" **(Acknowledge and respect).**

"We would like to hear the reason of not letting Miss C knowing her diagnosis, suppose First, we need to understand why family members may be hesitant to disclose a cancer diagnosis to the patient. In Chinese culture, there is a common belief that revealing a cancer diagnosis could negatively affect the patient's psychological well-being. This can often lead to a delay in diagnosis, which may further impact the patient's condition." **(Clarify).**

However, it is important not to completely conceal the cancer diagnosis. Understanding the diagnosis

and prognosis is essential for families to make informed decisions about advanced care planning and to set realistic expectations. We often recommend using more neutral terms, such as "abnormal cells," rather than directly stating "cancer" or "metastasis." Additionally, we may avoid explicitly discussing the stage of the disease or its incurable nature. **(Help).**

Our focus should be on reassuring the patient that the goal of the oncologists and healthcare providers is to alleviate symptoms and enhance quality of life. We encourage family members to gradually disclose the diagnosis to the patient over multiple consultations rather than all at once. Typically, our palliative care team can assist in facilitating this process, supporting the patient's needs and psychological well-being as they navigate the gradual progression of the disease. **(Help and engage).**

Decision Making and Ceiling of Medical Care in End-of-Life Care: The Role of Filial Piety

Filial Piety is a distinct behaviour of Chinese which emphasize for provision of care for the parents, and In the Confucian conceptualization it denotes "children's respect, obedience, and obligation to support their older parents emotionally and financially, honour ancestors, and preserve the family line through childbearing". The concept of filial piety will affect autonomy of patients for the advanced care planning in end-of-life care. Elaine Dabin Jeon et al., explores the dynamics of end-of-life care communication and decision-making in China, with a particular focus on the concepts of filial piety and the concealment of medical information by interviewing family and professional caregivers in 15 Chinese province.

Among all the interviews conducted, 26.9% (303 mentions) referenced filial piety, while 11.7% (86 mentions) addressed the concealment of medical information. The findings indicate that the autonomy of elderly patients is often compromised when family members, particularly adult children motivated by a strong sense of filial piety, control the disclosure of medical information and make decisions regarding end-of-life care.

Focusing Hong Kong as a metropolitan city with a mix of Chinese and Western culture, Cheng et al. studied the preferences for end-of-life care and decision-making among older adults living in the communities of Wuhan and Hong Kong. A cross-sectional correlational design was employed with convenience sample of 259 adults aged 65 years and older from five community centers in both cities.

The results revealed that participants from Wuhan were significantly more likely to view "trying every means to extend life" as very important or important. Additionally, they regarded "support from religious personnel" as unimportant or very unimportant. In contrast to their counterparts in Hong Kong, the older adults in Wuhan preferred to receive end-of-life care and to pass away in their own homes. Furthermore, they demonstrated a strong inclination for family members to take on the role of decision-makers in end-of-life situations.

Overall, it emphasizes the role of filial piety and the potential differences in preferences for end-of-life care and decision-making between older adults in Hong Kong and other province of China.

Progress of Mr. C's Condition – decision of Active Intervention in End-of-Life

Mr. C received treatment with EGFR-targeted therapy, which initially resulted in a very favorable clinical response. However, he subsequently experienced disease progression and was transitioned to palliative chemotherapy. Unfortunately, his condition further deteriorated in September 2024.

In September 2024, Mr. C was admitted to the oncology ward due to shortness of breath and became unresponsive as a result of respiratory failure. It was determined that he was experiencing respiratory failure due to hypoventilation. The medical team proposed the option of artificial ventilation, either through intubation or B Bi-level Positive Airway Pressure (BIPAP), which could potentially reverse hypercapnia and improve his level of consciousness. Given the sudden deterioration of his condition, Mr. C had not previously expressed his wishes regarding such interventions, according to his family members. A discussion took place among Mr. C's family regarding the choice between using Bi-level Positive Airway Pressure for respiratory support or opting for comfort care.

Progress of Mr. C

After extensive discussions with the family, a consensus was reached to initiate BIPAP to try for the reversal of hypercapnea. The family was informed.

- the primary goal is to reserve the hypercapnia, which may potentially improve the conscious level of the patient, allowing he to say the last goodbye words to the family members
- It was agreed that further escalation of artificial ventilation like intubation would not be considered if there was no clinical improvement after a trial of BIPA. Further use of inotropes
- Well acknowledged on the potential complications of BIPAP
- We aim to keep the consensus of DNACPR and wish to keep patients comfort as much as possible

Mr C received BIPAP and the conscious level improved after 2 days of BIPAP. He was able to communicate and say the goodbye words with his family in his late days. Eventually he deteriorated again due to shock and passed away peacefully.

Third Case Study—Mr. W

Mr. Chow is a ninety-five-year-old gentleman who has never smoked or consumed alcohol. His medical history includes hypertension and a valvular replacement for which he has been on long-term warfarin therapy.

In terms of his oncological history, Mr. Chow was incidentally discovered to have a left pleural effusion during a chest X-ray, while he was hospitalized for an intra-abdominal hematoma resulting from over-warfarinization. Subsequent imaging with a computed tomography (CT) scan of the thorax in June 2021 revealed multiple mediastinal lymphadenopathies, left pleural metastases with effusion, and bone metastases. The family declined a bronchoscopic biopsy due to concerns about the risks involved. However, an EGFR liquid biopsy indicated an EGFR exon 19 deletion.

Mr. Chow was first evaluated by our oncology team during an in-patient consultation. At that time, he was hospitalized for pneumonia and required up to 6 L of oxygen. The family agreed to a "do not attempt cardiopulmonary resuscitation" (DNACPR) order. Fortunately, his chest infection responded well to antibiotics, and his oxygen requirements were reduced to 2 L.

Since his admission, Mr. Chow has been bedbound, presenting with an ECOG performance status of 4. He experiences mild shortness of breath and requires long-term oxygen therapy at 2 L. Additionally, he suffers from mild bilateral lower limb edema and has hypoalbuminemia with a level of 18 g/L. A 5 cm × 5 cm sacral bedsore was also noted, resulting from prolonged immobility.

From a psychosocial perspective, Mr. Chow previously lived with his wife and son until May 2021, when he was transferred to a nearby nursing home due to caregiving challenges. Due to his advanced age, he is not fully aware of his medical condition, with his son serving as the primary decision-maker regarding his treatment.

Although a formal referral to a palliative care team was not made, discussions about advance care planning were initiated with Mr. Chow's family. As Mr. Chow is demented and not able to discuss on the clinical condition, the patient's daughter would be the main decision maker. The DNACPR decision was well accepted and thoroughly understood among family members, who expressed a desire to minimize the patient's suffering and manage his symptoms, given his bedbound status. However, in view of the presence of EGFR mutations, a discussion on the use of EGFR targeted therapy for Mr. W has been made.

Initiation of Targeted Therapy at End of Life—Case of Mr W

The initiation of targeted therapy in end-of-life care has become increasingly common, particularly due to the accessibility and application of non-invasive diagnostic test like liquid biopsies in lung cancer. Targeted therapies can result in remarkable responses in patients with specific driver mutations and are generally considered less toxic than conventional cytotoxic treatments. Evidence suggests that conventional cytotoxic therapies can be harmful at the end of life, often delaying the transition to palliative care. However, the use of targeted therapy in these situations is less clearly defined, raising ethical concerns regarding its tolerability and accessibility.

While in the case of Mr W, the the key decision maker is the family, foundation of medical ethics is applied and is grounded in four principles: autonomy, beneficence, non-maleficence, and justice. Each of these principles plays a crucial role in decision-making processes, particularly in the context of Mr. W's case. Oncologists should take reference to the four prinicples as the framework for discussion of treatment options.

Autonomy

Autonomy refers to an individual's right to make decisions regarding their own healthcare. In Mr. W's case, however, his status as a 95-year-old with dementia complicates the feasibility of obtaining proper consent. Consequently, discussions about initiating targeted therapy were conducted with his family, as they are likely to have a clearer understanding of his wishes.

Beneficence

Beneficence entails acting in the best interest of the patient. High-quality phase III data from the FLAURA trial demonstrate a substantial response rate of 80% and a median progression-free survival of 17.2 months for osimertinib as first-line treatment for EGFR mutant non-small cell lung cancer (NSCLC). If the disease responds to this therapy, Mr. Chow's symptoms of shortness of breath could improve, thereby enhancing his overall quality of life and well-being.

Non-Maleficence

Non-maleficence is the principle of "do no harm." While there is a lack of robust data specifically for patients with poor performance status, osimertinib generally has mild and tolerable side effects. Most reported adverse effects are grade 1–2, with severe events occurring in less than 2% of patients. However, patients receiving targeted therapy may encounter more aggressive treatment approaches, late referrals to hospice care, and a lack of discussion surrounding prognosis. To uphold non-maleficence, sensitive and thorough discussions between clinicians and family members are essential.

Justice

Justice pertains to the fair allocation of resources. In Mr. W's situation, the cost of the drug was borne by his family rather than through government funding. Therefore, its use did not compromise the availability of resources for other patients or the healthcare system as a whole.

To further illustrate the principle of non-maleficence, a retrospective population-based study in Taiwan analyzed data from 42,678 NSCLC patients from 2005 to 2012. It found that 21.3% of these patients received targeted therapy within 30 days of death. Those prescribed targeted therapy near the end of life were significantly more likely to experience aggressive care, including multiple emergency department visits, extended hospitalizations, and late hospice referrals.

Another study from the U.S., conducted by Petrillo et al., which included 154 patients as part of a secondary analysis of a randomized trial on early palliative care in advanced lung cancer, found that patients receiving targeted therapy reported greater improvements over time, independent of palliative care. They also tended to discuss prognosis less frequently with their clinicians and were more likely to receive cancer-directed therapy in the last 14 days of life. These findings indicate that patients receiving targeted therapy experience different health care utilization patterns compared to those without targetable mutations.

These studies underscore the need for integrating palliative care for patients undergoing targeted therapy, especially those who are frail or have a limited life expectancy due to underlying comorbidities. Without this integration, there is a risk of unnecessary aggressive treatment, inadequate discussions about prognosis, and insufficient preparation for end-of-life care, all of which could negatively impact the patient's quality of life and raise ethical concerns regarding non-maleficence.

Progress of Mr W

After extensive discussions with the family, a consensus was reached to initiate treatment with the third-generation tyrosine kinase inhibitor (TKI) osimertinib, as it is known to be an effective and non-toxic option. The family was informed.

- the primary goal of this treatment was to alleviate Mr. W's dyspnea, although they were cautioned that significant improvements in his overall functional status might not be achieved, even if the disease responded positively.
- It was agreed that cessation of the targeted therapy would be considered if there was no clinical improvement after a trial period.
- Well acknowledged on the side effects of the drugs
- We aim to keep the consensus of DNACPR and wish to keep patients comfort as much as possible

Regrettably, after starting osimertinib, there was minimal clinical improvement, and Mr. Chow continued to require 1–2 L of oxygen. Serial chest X-rays over three weeks indicated a static left lung whiteout, despite a slight decrease in tumor markers, Unfortunately, his clinical condition deteriorated further, characterized by reduced oral intake and overall decline. Ultimately, Mr. Chow passed away three weeks after initiation of targeted therapy following a sudden cardiac arrest, and the wishes outlined in the DNACPR order were respected.

Conclusion

Communication regarding oncology in Chinese populations faces distinct challenges due to cultural differences from Western practices. In China, decision-making is often family-oriented throughout various stages of the oncology journey. This includes critical moments such as breaking bad news, discussing treatment options, and making decisions about active interventions like initiating systemic treatment or resuscitation during end-of-life care. Core values in Chinese culture, particularly **filial piety**, frequently take precedence over patient autonomy, which can influence clinical judgment and lead to less-than-optimal palliative care, especially in end-of-life situations. The emphasis on family responsibilities may result in patients not fully participating in discussions about their health or treatment choices. Despite these challenges, enhancing communication skills and adhering to medical ethics remain fundamental to effective interactions and improved patient care. By fostering better communication practices, healthcare providers can navigate these cultural complexities and ultimately deliver higher quality care to patients. to medical ethics remain fundamental to effective interactions and improved patient care. By fostering better communication practices, healthcare providers can navigate these cultural complexities and ultimately deliver higher quality care to patients.

Discussion Prompts

1. What specific cultural values shape how Chinese families manage communication around terminal illness, and how do they differ from Western approaches?
2. How does the ARCHES framework help clinicians address requests for non-disclosure of diagnoses from family members? What are its ethical strengths and limitations?
3. In the cases of Mr. C, Miss C, and Mr. W, how did family involvement influence treatment decisions, including end-of-life care and use of targeted therapies?
4. How do economic and systemic factors (e.g., public healthcare limitations, cost of treatments) complicate shared decision-making between families and oncologists in Hong Kong?
5. What role does filial piety play in shaping decision-making authority, and how should clinicians ethically navigate potential tensions between family duty and patient autonomy?

Reflection Questions

1. Have you ever experienced or witnessed a situation where a family member requested that bad news not be disclosed to a patient? What communication strategies were or could have been used?
2. How would you balance the ethical principles of autonomy, beneficence, and non-maleficence in a situation where a patient is unaware of their terminal condition?
3. Reflecting on the cultural concept of "a good death," how might your own cultural background or personal values influence your preferences for communication and care at the end of life?
4. In what ways can clinicians involve family members constructively while still preserving the dignity and rights of the patient, especially in emotionally charged or time-sensitive situations?
5. After reading this chapter, what changes would you consider implementing in your own communication practices when working with patients and families in multicultural oncology settings?

Chapter 9
End-Of-Life Care: Navigating Death, Dying, and Survivorship from a Clinician's Voice

Sunny Kong

Introduction

Effective communication in end-of-life care is vital, particularly when addressing the complex emotional and medical needs of patients and their families. This chapter explores real-world scenarios to illustrate the challenges and opportunities in providing compassionate, patient-centered care in oncology. Based on Dr. Sunny Kong's recollections, these stories highlight the importance of understanding cultural nuances, fostering hope, and enabling shared decision-making.

Case Study 1: End-of-Life Care–The Emotional Toll of a Young Couple

Mrs. X, married only a few years, faced the unimaginable as her husband, Mr. X, succumbed to complications from a brain tumor. Despite advanced medical interventions, including surgery and a tracheostomy, his condition deteriorated, leaving the couple in a state of suspended hope. The palliative care team was brought in to address frequent infections and seizures.

In this emotionally charged setting, the role of the caregiver, often overlooked, came to the forefront. Mrs. X bore the emotional and physical strain of her husband's illness, feeling isolated and burdened by guilt. "I feel responsible, like I could have done something," she shared, reflecting the immense weight of such situations on caregivers.

S. Kong (✉)
Department of Medicine, Hong Kong Buddhist Hospital, Hong Kong, China
e-mail: sunny.kong@ha.org.hk

J. Pun (ed.), *Teaching and Learning Oncology Communication*,
https://doi.org/10.1007/978-981-96-9474-7_9

Ultimately, the decision to transition Mr. X to hospice care was met with uncertainty but underscored the importance of addressing emotional and logistical concerns comprehensively.

Case Study 2: Survivorship-The Optimistic Approach of Miss S

Miss S's journey from chemotherapy-induced complications to recovery offered insights into resilience and coping strategies. She embraced her illness with openness and optimism, engaging in candid discussions with friends and seeking clarity without overloading herself with medical details.

Her narrative highlights a critical lesson: fostering a sense of agency and positivity can significantly impact the patient's emotional well-being, even in the face of lingering side effects.

Case Study 3: The Ethical Dilemma in Treatment Decisions–Mr. B's Reflection on Hope and Treatment

For Mr. B, metastatic lung cancer presented a harrowing journey of treatment and side effects. His question, "Do you think I should proceed with the chemo?" opened a dialogue on the balance between extending life and maintaining quality of life.

The profound impact of hope—both as a motivator and a source of suffering—emerged as a central theme. Silence and empathetic listening became tools for understanding his true desires and fears, underscoring the delicate nature of end-of-life decision-making.

Case Study 4: Breaking Bad News–Miss W's Struggle with Acceptance

Miss W's late-stage bowel cancer diagnosis revealed the challenges of delivering bad news in a culturally sensitive and compassionate manner. Confronted with her fears and the responsibility of preparing her young children for life without her, Miss W's case exemplifies the emotional complexities of such situations.

Engaging the family in transparent discussions allowed for shared understanding and support, enabling Miss W to spend her remaining time meaningfully with her loved ones.

Lessons Learned and Practical Recommendations.

- **Communication Strategies:** The ARCHES framework provides a structured approach to balancing cultural sensitivities with the patient's right to information.
- **Cultural Sensitivity:** Understanding the role of family dynamics and cultural values, such as filial piety, is crucial in tailoring care.
- **Patient Empowerment:** Fostering hope and agency through shared decision-making enhances patient and family satisfaction.

Chapter 10
Conclusion

Jack Pun and Kexin Tan

In this book, we have comprehensively examined the multifaceted nature of oncology communication within the Chinese context, with a particular focus on Hong Kong. The chapters reveal the intricate interplay of traditional Chinese values, such as family-centric decision-making and the cultural reluctance to openly discuss death, with contemporary medical practices. These insights underscore the urgency of developing culturally sensitive communication strategies that align with the unique needs of patients and families navigating the complexities of cancer care.

From the outset, we recognized the cultural taboo against discussing death, as elaborated in Chapter 2. This reluctance often complicates discussions about prognosis, advanced care planning (ACP), and end-of-life care. We highlighted the pivotal role of family members, who frequently act as intermediaries in decision-making, contrasting with the patient autonomy emphasized in Western healthcare models. The chapter emphasized the need for healthcare providers to respect these familial dynamics while actively involving all stakeholders in the care process to ensure informed and compassionate decision-making.

Chapter 3 explored the professional identity construction of oncologists within the Chinese cultural framework. It examined how sociocultural norms and interprofessional collaboration influence their roles and practices, emphasizing the need for ongoing research to enhance understanding and support for oncologists as they navigate the challenges of oncology communication in this context.

The critical task of delivering bad news, addressed in Chapter 4, highlighted the importance of adapting the SPIKES protocol to fit Chinese cultural norms. Effective

J. Pun (✉)
Department of English, The Chinese University of Hong Kong, Hong Kong SAR, China
e-mail: jackpun@cuhk.edu.hk

K. Tan
Department of English and Communication, The Hong Kong Polytechnic University, Hong Kong SAR, China
e-mail: kexin.tan@connect.polyu.hk

J. Pun (ed.), *Teaching and Learning Oncology Communication*,
https://doi.org/10.1007/978-981-96-9474-7_10

communication strategies that incorporate linguistic subtleties and cultural competence were shown to be essential in navigating the tension between family traditions and patient preferences. This adaptation fosters compassionate care while respecting cultural values. Chapter 5 delves into the challenges and methodologies of comforting cancer patients in emotionally fraught situations. Through narrative practice, it highlights how providing a safe space for patients to share their stories can empower them to navigate their distress while fostering resilience. This chapter also addresses the emotional toll on healthcare providers, emphasizing the importance of setting boundaries, managing emotional labor, and acknowledging the potential for burnout. It advocates for mutual empowerment in clinician-patient interactions and stresses the need for training healthcare professionals to handle complex emotional scenarios with compassion and respect.

Chapter 6 delved into the role of end-of-life communication in palliative care. It underscored the necessity of open, culturally informed dialogues to clarify treatment expectations and ensure a "good death" characterized by dignity and peace. The chapter emphasized the challenges healthcare providers face in balancing explicit medical guidance with cultural sensitivities, advocating for strategies that honor both medical and cultural needs. In Chapter 7, the intricacies of prognostication were explored through the lens of Chinese palliative care. The dual processes of "foreseeing" and "foretelling" require not only medical accuracy but also a nuanced understanding of cultural values and ethical considerations. The chapter revealed that relational dynamics often take precedence over individual concerns, reflecting the collective search for meaning and understanding in confronting terminal illness. Finally, Chapters 8 and 9 delve into the pivotal role of clinicians in oncology communication, focusing on family dynamics and end-of-life care within the Chinese cultural context. Through detailed case studies, these chapters explore how clinicians navigate the complexities of breaking bad news, treatment planning, and decision-making in end-of-life scenarios. Chapter 8 highlights the clinician's role in managing family involvement, emphasizing the importance of culturally sensitive communication strategies such as the ARCHES framework. This framework helps balance respecting family preferences with the patient's right to information, fostering trust and collaboration. Chapter 9 complements this perspective by addressing the emotional, ethical, and cultural challenges inherent in end-of-life care, illustrating how tailored communication can empower patients and families. Together, these chapters underscore the necessity of equipping healthcare providers with the skills to navigate these sensitive dynamics while honoring the cultural values of patients and their families. As we conclude, this book calls for concerted efforts from healthcare professionals, policymakers, and community leaders to prioritize cultural competence in oncology communication. By embracing culturally sensitive approaches and fostering interdisciplinary collaboration, we can pave the way for more compassionate and effective cancer care in the Chinese context.

Call to Action for Chinese Stakeholders

To realise this vision, we need to mobilise action from a range of stakeholders in China's health system. Here are specific steps that professionals, policymakers and community leaders can take:

First, health professionals must improve their training by integrating cultural competence and communication skills into both medical education and continuing education. This includes workshops that focus on family dynamics and traditional beliefs about death and dying, enabling providers to engage more effectively with patients and their families. Also, the development of resources such as the proposed 'Compassionate Communication Guide' could greatly assist in navigating difficult conversations and ensure that healthcare providers are well-equipped to support their patients.

At the same time, policymakers have a critical role to play in implementing guidelines that promote culturally sensitive communication practices in all healthcare settings. Establishing national standards that emphasise family involvement and the need for clear, compassionate dialogue can provide a framework within which healthcare providers can operate. In addition, investing in research initiatives that examine the impact of culturally sensitive communication on patient outcomes will inform policy decisions and healthcare practices nationwide.

Community leaders also have an important role to play in promoting public engagement. By organising community forums and workshops that encourage open discussions about cancer care, death and dying, these leaders can help normalise conversations about end-of-life issues. Such initiatives empower families to articulate their wishes and experiences, thereby strengthening community bonds and the overall support system.

In addition, academic institutions should encourage interdisciplinary collaboration between medical schools, social work programmes and cultural studies departments. This collaboration can lead to the creation of comprehensive training programmes that address the social and cultural aspects of healthcare communication, ensuring that future healthcare professionals are well-prepared to navigate the complexities of their roles.

As we move forward, let us commit to a future where every conversation in oncology is infused with compassion and cultural awareness. By taking these actionable steps, we can cultivate a healthcare environment that not only respects but celebrates the diverse tapestry of cultural values that shape the patient experience. Together, we can ensure that every patient and family feels empowered, supported and dignified throughout their cancer journey. Let this serve as a catalyst for ongoing dialogue, research, and practice improvement in oncology communication.

Discussion Prompts

1. How do traditional Chinese cultural values influence the communication strategies discussed throughout the book? What common patterns emerged across chapters?

2 Why is it important to incorporate cultural competence into medical education, and how can interdisciplinary collaboration enhance this training?
3 What roles do various stakeholders—health professionals, policymakers, community leaders, and academics—play in promoting culturally sensitive oncology communication?
4 How can communication models like SPIKES and ARCHES be adapted to better reflect family-oriented decision-making in Chinese settings?
5 In what ways can the proposed 'Compassionate Communication Guide' support clinicians facing emotionally charged and culturally complex scenarios?

Reflection Questions

1 Reflect on your personal or professional context: How culturally responsive is your current approach to healthcare communication? What might you change after reading this chapter?
2 What challenges do you foresee in implementing national guidelines that promote culturally sensitive communication, and how might these be addressed?
3 Which chapter(s) influenced your thinking the most about end-of-life care, and why? How might these insights affect your future practice or teaching?
4 How can open conversations about death and dying be normalized in traditionally reserved cultures? What role can you play in this shift?
5 After engaging with this book, how has your understanding of 'a good death' or patient-centered care evolved in the context of Chinese cultural values?

Correction to: A Narrative Approach to Comfort

Weiwei Lu

Correction to:
Chapter 5 in: J. Pun (ed.), *Teaching and Learning Oncology Communication*, https://doi.org/10.1007/978-981-96-9474-7_5

The original version of the book was inadvertently published with error in chapter 5 pages 61, 62, 64. Strikethrough text were retained in page 62 and 64. This has been corrected.

The updated version of this chapter can be found at
https://doi.org/10.1007/978-981-96-9474-7_5

J. Pun (ed.), *Teaching and Learning Oncology Communication*,
https://doi.org/10.1007/978-981-96-9474-7_11

Index

J. Pun (ed.), *Teaching and Learning Oncology Communication*,
https://doi.org/10.1007/978-981-96-9474-7

M

N

O

P

MIX
Papier aus verantwortungsvollen Quellen
Paper from responsible sources
FSC® C105338

If you have any concerns about our products,
you can contact us on
ProductSafety@springernature.com

In case Publisher is established outside the EU,
the EU authorized representative is:
Springer Nature Customer Service Center GmbH
Europaplatz 3, 69115 Heidelberg, Germany

Printed by Libri Plureos GmbH
in Hamburg, Germany